Healing Foods

Healing Foods

How to nurture yourself and fight illness

DR ROSY DANIEL

The Bristol Cancer Help Centre

Thorsons
An Imprint of HarperCollins*Publishers*

Thorsons
An Imprint of HarperCollins*Publishers*
77–85 Fulham Palace Road,
Hammersmith, London W6 8JB

1160 Battery Street,
San Francisco, California 94111-1213

Published by Thorsons 1996

10 9 8 7 6 5 4 3 2 1

A catalogue record for this book
is available from the British Library

ISBN 0 7225 3280 6

Printed and bound in Great Britain by
Caledonian International Book Manufacturing Ltd, Glasgow

This book is dedicated to Seventy Smith, Katrina Collins and Beata Bishop – just three of the many people who have shown me that cancer can regress through healthy eating alone; to the transformation of the health of the western world as we properly embrace the reality of the impact of our food on our health; and to the recovery of our planet as we relearn how to grow organic whole food which truly nourishes life without damaging the environment.

Contents

Acknowledgements

I would like to express my gratitude to the pioneers of the healthy approach to eating at the Bristol Cancer Help Centre, and above all to acknowledge the vision, dedication and generosity of those who created the centre and for whom my admiration knows no bounds – Penny Brohn, Pat and Christopher Pilkington, and Dr Alec Forbes, and our original nutritional therapist Ute Brookman who remains at the Centre to this day. I would also like to acknowledge my heartfelt thanks to my wonderful, generous-hearted assistant Caroline Morrison, who has supported me and helped me tirelessly through the process of producing this book; to my lovely editor Wanda Whiteley for her faith and encouragement in the project, and to Barbara Vesey and the production team at Thorsons for their great work. My love and thanks also go to my husband John and my children, who have supported me through the writing of the book, and put up with my temporary absence. Thank you all for your help with this important work.

Foreword

We are what we eat. How many times have we all heard that simple health education message and ignored its impact? Through aeons of evolutionary time, we as a race have survived and developed. But over the last 50 years, two sudden and major changes have taken place. We can now live much longer thanks to medical science, and this trend continues. But increasing affluence and new food technology – production, storage and preparation – has led to the average Western diet becoming distinctly unhealthy. This combination of increased life expectancy and a poor diet is leading to an unprecedented epidemic of potentially lethal diseases such as cancer, heart attacks and strokes. It has been estimated that 35 per cent of cancers are caused by an unhealthy diet, as are about 50 per cent of arterial disease. So what can we do about it? We need two things: motivation and information. This is where this very timely book by Rosy Daniel comes in.

Here you will find some very practical advice. We in Britain are overfed with the wrong sorts of food – produced by an industry that spends millions of pounds each year on slick advertising and marketing strategies. A healthy diet need not be expensive. This easy to read guide tells you how to change your diet for the better.

The first chapter tells you why you should change your diet. Reducing total calorie intake to avoid obesity is an obsession with many, but it's *what* we eat as well as how much that is important. Dieting and bingeing are often written about, but are irrelevant to the long-term change in diet required to be healthy. The second chapter tells you how to make the necessary change to your diet; the third chapter details what to change.

There is still much uncertainty about our food and its relationship to health. A small amount of alcohol may, for example, be beneficial. Eating lean meat may also be useful and is an excellent source of protein. But four principles, stressed time and again in this book, come over strongly in all serious studies of the subject:

1 reduce your intake of animal fat;
2 increase your daily fibre content;
3 eat plenty of fresh fruit and vegetables;
4 avoid obesity.

The fourth chapter concludes this book with the concept of food as therapy. There is no doubt that conventional medicine has fastidiously avoided this area. Evidence of objective benefit is difficult to evaluate. But if a patient can feel better by changing his or her diet, then by definition this change has a positive effect. Increasingly, people with a wide range of illnesses want to experiment with their diet – it is part of the empowering process that puts the patient in the driving seat. This book provides some very safe and sound advice for us all.

Karol Sikora PhD, FRCR, FRCP, Professor of Clinical Oncology, Royal Postgraduate Medical School, Hammersmith Hospital, and Deputy Director, Imperial Cancer Research Fund, London

Introduction

Back in the early 1980s, Dr Alec Forbes – who was at that time Medical Director of the Bristol Cancer Help Centre – published a book called *The Bristol Diet*. This 'anti-cancer diet' was the synthesis of his own views, the views of our nutritional therapist Ute Brookman, and elements from the Gerson Diet. Many of those who came to the Bristol Cancer Help Centre, and even many who did not, tried this diet with great success. These people reported a very rapid improvement in their energy and in the condition of their skin, hair, nails and digestive processes. Many reported that after 6 to 12 weeks on the diet they felt clearer mentally and better in their bodies than they had felt for years. These reports were followed by observations that the side-effects of radiotherapy and chemotherapy decreased, and a significant number of people felt that they were witnessing a regression of their cancer.

On the other hand there were others who found the diet extremely stressful, who lost weight and whose doctors understandably felt very critical about the Bristol Diet. The stress arose from a sense of failure if the diet could not be strictly adhered to, combined with the struggle to shop for, prepare and cook the required amounts of juices, salads and vegan meals. In some cases weight loss resulted from an excessive focus by individuals on eating too much raw food without taking in enough starch and calories to maintain their normal weight.

After the departure of Dr Forbes in 1985, the Centre's approach to food was reviewed and what was devised was 'the healthy approach to eating', which comprised a wholefood diet high in vegetables, fruit, cereals and pulses, and low in animal fats, protein, salt and sugar. What has been realized is that where food and cancer are concerned there is a spectrum of options with food as therapy at one end and healthy eating at the other. It is also clear that the 'food as therapy' approach is extremely good for those whom it suits temperamentally and physically, but that it is wrong to 'prescribe' this approach for everyone. The Cancer Help Centre would still support individuals wishing to choose a rigorous dietary approach such as the Bristol Diet, Gerson Diet or perhaps naturopathic or macrobiotic diets to fight their cancer. However, what is recommended to all who come is a gradual shift to a very healthy, balanced, nutritious diet which is as suitable for the prevention of cancer as for the promotion of health and strength in those who are fighting cancer.

The truth of the matter is that this is the sort of diet which all of us in the West should be moving towards. We know that cancer, arterial disease and probably rheumatoid arthritis, asthma and diabetes all have extremely strong dietary links, and that the main culprits are our excessive consumption of animal foods and sugary and processed foods. The problem is that although most of us know this we are often very resistant to making the change to a healthy diet.

This resistance may be put down to a number of factors. Obviously there is the pleasure that we all take in consuming rich, sweet foods. There is great comfort in the instant gratification that we can get from sweets, chocolates and takeaway fried foods. There is the social pressure to conform and all the pressure on women to be good home-makers and mothers and to produce food to win the approval and affection of loved ones. And, of course, there is the negative image surrounding healthy food. How often have we heard it described as 'rabbit food', 'hippy food', or being equated with total deprivation!

This means that there are two major tasks to be achieved. The first is to show people how to change their diet in such a way that the change is sustainable and permanent and does not result in a feeling of failure or getting into a dieting and bingeing cycle. The second is to change the image of this way of eating altogether.

The first of these objectives is my reason for writing this book, which I hope will serve as an extremely practical guide both to those with cancer and to those wishing to achieve positive health in order to prevent a whole range of 'Western' illnesses. The second of these objectives is tackled by our inspired new chef, Jane Sen, in her *Healing Foods Cookbook*. Jane has come to the Cancer Help Centre from a background at the highest level of international *haute cuisine*, and has brought her immense creativity and skill to bear on revolutionizing the image of healthy food. Her *Healing Foods Cookbook* will herald the launch of her new cooking style, 'Cuisine Vivante'.

We hope that, armed with both books, you will have the knowledge, guidance, support and inspiration to embark upon a new style of cooking and eating. This change will not only bring you good health but also be a wonderful outlet for your creativity and a great source of pleasure.

CHAPTER ONE

Why Change the Way You Eat?

THE EFFECTS OF OUR WESTERN DIET

It is now time that all of us who eat a typical Western diet should be making the move to change the way we eat. Cancer and arterial disease (which causes heart attacks and strokes) are most strongly associated with our unhealthy eating patterns; people from Japan, China and Africa who take up a Western lifestyle and diet quickly start to demonstrate the same vulnerability to these lethal illnesses, having previously been protected by their more balanced diet.

Cancer and arterial disease now kill 75 per cent of British people – the highest rate anywhere in the world.[1]

Our Diet is Badly Out of Proportion

An unhealthy diet causes 35 per cent of cancer in the Western world, even more than does smoking, which causes 30 per cent of our cancer.[2] The problem is that our diet has evolved faster than our bodies' ability to cope with it. As we have grown more afflu-ent our diet has become richer in both fats and proteins, and has become more highly flavoured with salt, sugar, spices and addi-tives. Simultaneously, food has become far more processed and refined, its valuable roughage and nutrients being taken out. We have also tended to eat fewer and fewer vegetables, cereals, pulses and fruits. The end result is a bizarre paradox whereby we are both overfed *and* undernourished, with a resulting chronic deteri-oration in our energy levels and in the body's immune system and ability to repair itself, and a generalized increase in our suscepti-bility to disease.

In China, fat consumption makes up 13 per cent of the diet, as compared with 40 per cent in the UK; animal proteins account for only 7 per cent of all protein eaten as compared with 70 per cent in the UK, and coronary heart disease is lower by a ratio of 4:100 in China than the UK (that is, for every four heart disease suffer-ers in China, there are 100 in the UK).[3]

> Vegetarians are 40 per cent less likely to die from cancer[4] and 30 per cent less likely to die from cardiovascular disease.[5]

Excess Food and Energy Depletion

The chronic excess of fat, protein, salt and sugar puts the body into a state of physiological stress and toxicity. This happens because our systems are designed in such a way that we can only tolerate a very small variation in the levels of these substances within our blood, otherwise the functioning of many of our deli-cate tissues, particularly the brain, goes haywire. In order to regu-late the blood levels of these substances, the liver, kidney and pancreas have to work extremely hard. Not only do these processes cost the body a great deal of energy, but they also use up valuable minerals, vitamins and enzymes, depleting the body stores of these vital substances as a result. This exaggerates the depletion we already suffer as a result of our nutritionally impoverished diets.

In the short term the effects of this process can be recognized by the drowsiness and nausea we may feel following a rich meal, which may inhibit our ability to function properly for an hour or two afterwards. But more sinister than this is the effect on our energy over the long term. The most common complaint faced by GPs nowadays is the new TATT syndrome: 'Tired All The Time'! Of course, we get into a vicious cycle here because the lethargy created by bad eating habits disinclines us to exercise properly, and this, coupled with sedentary jobs, stress and other bad habits such as drinking and smoking, precipitate us into a state of chronic exhaustion.

Body Breakdown

The problem does not stop here! Despite its best efforts the body rarely can completely metabolize and excrete away the excess fat, protein, sugar and salt, so oftentimes its only recourse is to store these substances inappropriately in the cells or in deposits along the lining of the blood vessels themselves. This in turn leads to hardening of the arteries, fluid retention due to the ensuing imbalance of sodium, potassium and glucose in the cells, and even the depositing of proteins within the tissues (which may well contribute to antibody production and auto-immune processes, where the body starts to make antibodies against itself as occurs in such diseases as rheumatoid arthritis).

In these conditions no tissues of the body can work well, and functioning at all levels becomes compromised; we also become fat and prone to cellulite, varicose veins, skin problems and long-term stress on our musculo-skeletal system. The skin itself is an organ of excretion, and many of the greasy skin problems and ensuing spots we suffer from in the West (for which we are sold billions of pounds' worth of cosmetics each year) arise from the skin playing its part in excreting excess fats and toxins. The effect of excess on the musculo-skeletal system is obviously seen in increased wear and tear on the system and the degenerative disease of osteoarthritis. The general stiffness many of us experience without actually having joint disease is also due to these deposits of excess fat, protein, sugar and salt.

Gut Disorders
Further to this we have more problems created by the fact that we do not eat enough fibre, fruit, vegetables, cereals or pulses. The primary effect of this deficiency is on our bowel. The passage of food through the body is slowed down, which often leads to discomfort, abdominal distension, constipation and piles, and sometimes irritable bowel syndrome and diverticulitis. The secondary effect is that the slow transit time of food through the gut leaves far longer for any toxins present within food to be absorbed. It has been found that those on high-fibre diets who accidentally take in toxins or bacteria often stay well, while those on low-fibre diets get stomach upsets.

Food Absorption
It takes several hours to digest the cellulose-bound nutrients in fruits, cereals, pulses and vegetables, meaning that after this type

of meal there is a gentle trickle of nutrients into the body over a period of many hours. When a very concentrated sugary or fatty food is eaten in a very easily digestible form, such as glucose in a chocolate bar or fat coating a fried meal, this moves very quickly into the bloodstream, causing an enormous peak in the levels of sugar and fat in the blood which have to be removed very quickly by the liver and pancreas. This results in the rapid change from a large peak in blood levels to a trough in the blood levels of these substances. This often creates irritability and more hunger, and a tendency to rush to other foods which may give quick gratification but again set off the vicious cycle described here.

Mucus Production

There is another marked effect of eating excess fat and protein, particularly as a result of a large intake of dairy foods: the production of a great deal of excess mucus – yet another way the body attempts to excrete the excess. This in turn leads to a tendency to infection, rheumatic illnesses and exacerbation of allergies. It might interest you to know that the Chinese word for cheese is 'solid mucus' – Needless to say, milk products form a very small part of the traditional Chinese diet!

Vitamin and Mineral Deficiency

Of course, the other big problem about our low intake of fruits, vegetables, cereals and pulses is that these foods form the major source of vitamins and, particularly, minerals. These plant foods also have high levels of *essential fatty acids*, which are far better for us than the type of fatty acids found in meat. They are also rich in plant enzymes, which have a highly beneficial effect on our metabolic, growth and repair processes. The definition of the word 'vitamin' is 'vital for life' – need I say more?

Another phenomenon which occurs in the West is that our appetites can be subdued by foods which have plenty of calories but no nutritional value. For example, a chocolate bar may completely satisfy us but it has virtually nothing other than sugar in it. To get the same number of calories we would have to eat around 2 kilos (5 lb) of apples; in the process we would also have given ourselves a huge amount of valuable vitamins, minerals, fibre and enzymes. This brings us back to the idea of being overfed and undernourished simultaneously.

All of the vitamins, minerals and essential fatty acids required by our bodies are vital for the correct functioning of our tissues. It is now clear that vitamins A, C, and E (sometimes known as the antioxidant vitamins), in combination with the minerals zinc and selenium, play an especially important role in protecting us against cancer by de-activating dangerous *free radicals* – chemicals taken into and formed in the body as a result of pollution and dietary impurities. Free radicals attack lipids, proteins, enzymes and DNA, causing a variety of pathological events and cancer. Vitamins are vital to protect the cells and to keep the cancer-producing 'free radical' chemicals produced by chemical carcinogens, radiation and the metabolic stress of an unhealthy diet from causing *oxidative damage* and transforming into cancer cells.

The recommended daily allowances of these substances as quoted by the medical profession are the amounts required to keep us free from deficiency diseases such as scurvy and rickets – we need far more to maintain positive health, however. A large proportion of our diet should be made up of fruit and vegetables, especially as petrochemical, insecticide and fertilizer pollution worsens. Many people now take these substances (in the form of vitamin/mineral supplements) regularly as a preventive; details of

using vitamins and minerals in prevention and treatment are given in Chapter 4 of this book.

It seems that we have a great myth to break – that the more we eat, especially in terms of all those things that were once thought to be especially good for us, like milk, cheese, butter, cream and meat – the healthier we will be. In fact it is clear that the reverse is true, and that it is essential that we return to a diet far closer in nature to that of the poorer countries of the world, based predominantly on carbohydrates, pulses, nuts, vegetables and fruits, with a far lower intake of protein, fat and food additives.

THE QUALITY OF FOOD IN 'CIVILIZED' SOCIETY

Unfortunately, the disproportion of our Western diet is not the only problem. There is also the huge issue of how our food is produced, processed, packaged and stored, and hence what sort of shape it is in by the time it reaches our kitchens.

Intensive Farming
Most farmers have been forced through economic pressures into extremely intensive farming processes where high yield is achieved with chemicals, fertilizers and hormones which speed growth and add bulk.

Agriculture
Because of the pressure to produce crop after crop of vegetables out of the same land, there is a breakdown in the health and homeostasis of the soil, meaning that yet more chemicals are

used to control diseases, pests and weeds. On a lettuce farm where I once worked through a summer holiday, the same piece of earth was used over and over again, new plants being planted within hours of the old ones being cut. For each crop the soil was sprayed six times – twice with weed killers, twice with pesticides, and twice with fertilizers. The more toxic pesticides were sprayed onto the bare soil, directly adjacent to young plants which were already growing and could not possibly have avoided contamination. This chemical onslaught occurs before the second round of sprays, gases and radiation used to keep fruit and vegetables perfect in transit!

The overall effect of these practices is that often growth is too quick for the usual nutrients to develop and become incorporated into the plants; this problem is exacerbated because the soil is already low in the vital trace elements because of repeated usage. So the vegetables may look perfect but be tasteless, watery or even hollow inside in the case of some carrots; certainly they do not contain the nutrients we would expect to find in them. To boot, these vegetables have been found to contain the chemicals used to stimulate their growth and protect them from bugs. It is impossible to wash these substances off and avoid contamination ourselves with toxic chemicals (although careful washing will help remove chemicals used once the product has grown).

> Banning of organochlorine pesticide Lindane in Israel has brought the overall breast cancer incidence down by 8 per cent, and the rate in the lowest age group down by 24 per cent.[6]

Animal Husbandry

In animals, growth-stimulating factors such as steroids and hormones may be used to speed growth, add muscle bulk and increase milk and egg production. Drugs are also used to control pests and disease. As with humans, these practices weaken the ability of the animal to eradicate disease and infection. These substances may be found in high quantities within the meat and particularly liver of the animal, and of course may be passed at higher levels, dissolved in fat or through the animal's milk into dairy foods as the animal itself excretes the chemicals. (These substances become most concentrated in high-fat foods such as cheese and cream.) Added to this is the effect of contaminating pesticides and fertilizers on the grass the animals eat and in the feed and water they are given, which will also pass to humans through animal products – particularly those products high in fat.

There is another issue here, too: the potential for transmission of infection from animal food. Being far closer in our make-up to animals than to the plant kingdom, we are likely to be prone to similar infecting agents. Animal foods put us at risk of infection from bacteria such as salmonella (eggs), listeria (cheese), and viruses such as BSE from beef. These are the ones we know about – I feel sure many other of the mystery diseases of our time will be found to have their origins in infections transmitted in this way.

We see, therefore, that modern food production leaves us with food of a lower nutritional value which may also be quite polluted, toxic, infectious and antigenic. Many members of the older generation complain about the tastelessness of many of our vegetables, fruits and meats, and the way that bulk-produced chicken even tastes of fish (it is often fed on fish meal). Indeed, anyone who has ever had a garden of his or her own will be staggered by the difference in the taste of fresh homegrown vegetables compared with the beautiful but nutritionally pale imitations which are generally on offer in our shops.

Food Processing

Sadly, the processing of food which occurs to transform the raw material into highly marketable goodies of one sort or another further damages it by removing the fibre, roughage and essential nutrients. Much processing came about through the fashion of 'refining' food – turning brown flour white, brown rice white and brown sugar white. In the process many important vitamins, minerals and *co-factors* (required to promote the activity of other substances, such as vitamins) are lost. In addition to this there is further destruction of vitamins and enzymes in heating processes; the addition of chemicals in the processes of bleaching, dyeing, flavouring, emulsifying and stabilizing; not to mention the effects of plastic containers and *gamma-irradiation*. Plastic containers and bottles are believed to release potentially toxic chemicals into their contents, and nowadays many foods, especially fruits, vegetables and spices, are irradiated to prevent decay. Little is known as yet about the potential dangers of this practice.

However, what becomes clear when we look at the frighteningly long sell-by dates on many packaged and processed foods is that the foods have been rendered virtually inert nowadays. It is very much in the producers' interests to control all the normal decaying processes, but the risk is that the life is knocked completely out of the food and we are left with a chemical corpse rather than a living, vibrant, natural food. The most vivid illustration of this can be seen using Kirlian photography, which shows us visually the vital energy radiating from matter. An organic brown loaf has an energy field several centimetres deep, whereas a white processed loaf has no energy field at all!

We may go on to add insult to injury in the types of cooking methods we use. For example, frying foods at very high temperatures tends to de-nature them, as most enzymes and vitamins cannot withstand high temperatures. In the process, dangerous and unstable free radicals are produced in the fat and in the food being cooked. Even worse is barbecuing, when the presence of *hydrocarbons* in the smoke accelerates this process, especially in the cooking of meat. The curing of meat with *salt petre* (as in many salamis) is also dangerous because the sodium nitrite can change to carcinogenic nitrosamines in the gut.

Microwaving food may have similarly destructive effects, as microwaves are extremely high energy and heat the food even hotter than most frying techniques. This is why microwaved foods must always be left to stand after microwaving, as otherwise the high energy will be dissipated in our gullet and stomach with potentially dangerous consequences. Freezing food is not intrinsically so bad, however food does deteriorate in the freezer over time and the freezer should not be used to store food for months and months.

The net result of modern-day food production, therefore, is that it provides us with food which may look wonderful but which may be more dead than alive, lacking in nutrients, contaminated with chemicals and growth factors, and with a very low fibre content to boot.

Water

It is also likely that the water we drink from our taps may be seriously contaminated. Many water authorities do not yet routinely measure for byproducts produced by the plastics, petrochemical and farming industries. Organochlorines, for example, may mimic hormones and could possibly be responsible for the dramatic rise in hormone-related cancers (most commonly lung, breast and prostate). Of course, foods and water may be being pronounced safe, but this is only valid when the presence of contaminants is known about and measured, when the effects of these contaminants are known, and of course when those with a commercial interest do not suppress the distribution of information!

THE QUANTITY OF FOOD WE EAT

Most of us in the West simply eat far too much. Over 60 per cent of British adults are overweight, and the proportion is even higher in the US. In fact, it has been said that the amount spent on slimming products in the richer countries of the world could easily solve the problem of starvation in Third World countries. Our hunger can be satisfied with relatively modest amounts of food, but we go on and on eating for all sorts of other reasons. This would not be so bad if the foods we were eating were high in fibre and low in calories, but usually the reverse is true. Obviously the obesity created is a problem. It makes us less mobile and far less inclined to exercise. This in turn renders us more sluggish, with accompanying deterioration of our posture. Joints suffer and the tendency to arthritic problems is aggravated. We are also put at risk of high blood-pressure and poor circulation, and become an anaesthetic risk if we require surgery.

We are also afflicted by the damage to our self-image that being fat creates, and carry the further burden of stress, dieting and bingeing. On top of all these well-known problems of obesity is the newer association which is being made between obesity and cancer risk. Originally it was noted anecdotally that women in P.O.W. camps on poor diets had almost no breast cancer. The relationship between high calorie intake and cancer of the breast, prostate, colon and ovary has since been demonstrated. Animal studies have shown that a reduction in food intake by 30 per cent stopped all tumour growth altogether and doubled the life expectancy of the animals. Further animal studies have shown that decreasing the amounts of protein, sugar and fat in the diet reduces tumour growth directly and exponentially.

While it has been almost impossible to repeat these studies on humans (as it is hard to expect a randomized group to remain on a low-calorie diet for long periods of time in order to measure the possible effect on tumour development), it has certainly become clear that fat is strongly associated with many cancers, particularly the hormonal cancers (breast, ovary, uterus, prostate, testicular), and also colon cancer. The association is far stronger with animal fats than vegetable fats, and the overall incidence of cancer is much higher in the rich countries than the poor ones. Fat is seen not as initiating cancer, but as promoting it once it exists in the body.

> The American Cancer Society say that the overweight have a 50 per cent higher incidence of cancer.

Drink
Sweetened drinks and alcohol are a major source of extra calories and obesity in the West. Twenty years ago most people drank water with their meals, and alcohol or sweetened drinks were

reserved for special occasions. Nowadays it is not uncommon for individuals to take in an extra 1,000 calories a day through fizzy 'pop', beer, wine and spirits, mixers, and the milk and sugar in tea and coffee. Again we are in the trap of 'empty calories' – becoming satisfied by substances with almost no nutritional value, and making ourselves fat in the process.

It is known that fatty tissue produces hormones, and it may well be through this mechanism alone that being overweight creates extra cancer risk. Alternatively, as mentioned before, it may be due to risk factors present in the animal fats we are taking in either directly in meat or through dairy produce. Animal fat contains both the animal's own hormones and other growth-stimulating substances used to promote its growth and milk production, or chemicals ingested from feeds, grass or water. In short, both the animal's fat and our own fat become manufacturers and stores of potentially harmful substances which are putting us at higher risk of cancer. It is worth pointing out here that the fat in chicken and fish, unlike that in other meats, is stored more exclusively under the skin than in the flesh, so it is easier to eliminate before cooking (by removing and discarding the skin) if desired.

HOW WE EAT

Next we must face the question of how we eat and therefore how able we are to digest our food and gain nutritional benefit from it. In order to digest and absorb food properly, we must be relaxed. When we are stressed, rushed or preoccupied with other things, our nervous system is in a state of arousal. This favours the operation of our brain and muscles – in other words the organs of doing and thinking, fight and flight. This happens at the expense of the internal housekeeping functions of the body, which cannot work optimally unless we are in a relaxed state and the 'attention' of our organism can be directed into digestion, absorption, metabolism, immune function, growth and repair. This means that we can be eating quite good food but only be getting a small proportion of its nutritional benefits. An extreme example of this is seen in the failure-to-thrive syndrome in babies, where their growth is inhibited by the fear and anxiety they suffer as a result of lack of physical contact, bonding and love. In this state, absorption of food and actual growth come to a virtual standstill.

In our stressed, rushed 20th century lifestyles when many meals are eaten on the hoof, in the car, while talking on the telephone and doing 20 other things, our digestion and nutrition are severely compromised. Whether we stop to eat and enjoy our food or not can become one of the clearest signs of whether we are literally able to give ourselves space and time to nourish ourselves at the physical level, let alone emotionally and spiritually.

Comfort Eating
Food is very commonly used as an emotional prop, both for comfort and to take away difficult feelings – by eating or not eating. For some a sense of control in life is re-established through the withholding of food, sometimes to the point of anorexia. Rich, sweet and fatty foods have a sedative effect on us because of their toxicity and the work which the body has to do to re-establish equilibrium. Food for some may therefore be taking the place of tranquillizers! Many people discover when they try to change their diet, omitting the unhealthier foods, that they are suddenly

faced with emotions and feelings which they have been suppressing for years and with which they feel unable to cope.

This sort of situation can lead to addictive dependency on food in just the same sort of way people become dependent on drink or drugs. It can even sometimes be seen that people become addicted to foods to which they are actually quite allergic, because the symptoms and drowsiness they experience while their body is dealing with the challenge relieves them temporarily of some of their anxiety or other painful feelings. This can be exploited by others, who can control them through 'comfort feeding'. Many people keep their families dependent on and attached to them, trading unconsciously on the power of control that over-feeding gives them.

Social Eating

Another distorting factor in the relationship between what we eat and what our bodies need is the extensive use of food in social situations. Most entertaining revolves almost exclusively around food and drink, and often party food is almost entirely made up of pastries, cakes, crisps, biscuits, and fried and barbecued foods, all washed down with large amounts of very sweet fizzy drinks and alcohol. In these types of situations we may be taking in our calorific requirement for several days in one sitting!

Eating in restaurants is the most common leisure-time activity, and of course fast food is always available on the street, at home, or delivered to your door at all hours of the night and day. To make things worse, often the insecure host or hostess will aim to please, and go on feeding guests more and more, using food as an entertainment or as a way of augmenting a lack of social skills! By far the majority of food which is eaten in social contexts has nothing at all to do with our nutritional needs, and forms a great part of the distorting influence on our health and lifestyle in the late 20th century.

Eating Patterns Through the Day

As well as the problem of eating our food fast while we are preoccupied, there is a growing tendency to leave the largest meal until very late in the day. Often breakfast is reduced to a cup of coffee, and lunch a quick sandwich; dinner becomes the serious meal of the day. This plays havoc with the metabolism of the body, because during the part of the day when we have the biggest need for energy, energy is having to be produced from stored substances such as glycogen and fat. Whereas at night, when we are sleeping, the body is being flooded with available energy sources from the large meal we have just eaten. It would appear that the problem with this is that not only is the work of storing and liberating the energy-producing nutrients being done twice, but that we end up storing more than we use. This is because at times of very low blood sugar during the day the body moves into very efficient metabolic mode, liberating as little of the stored tissue as it can. The net result is that we gain weight, as more and more food will be laid down during the night as fat, and less will be changed back during the day for available energy supply.

It is therefore very important that we revert to either the more continental habit of eating the main meal at midday, with only a snack during the evening; or to the traditional Eastern habit of having the largest meal at breakfast time. Of course, again, the prime requirement here is that we slow down and once again make eating an important part of our day.

Dieting and Bingeing – Fighting Fashion

One of the greatest jokes of our time is that despite the fact that 60 per cent of society is overweight, fashion continues to portray the image of lean, firm-fleshed, healthy looking slim people as the ideal towards which we must all strive. In fact many models are so thin that they are clearly bordering on anorexia. This would seem to point to the underlying revulsion we feel with our out-of-control bodies and eating habits. The media clearly taps into and exploits this self-hatred, perpetually encouraging us to invest in clothes, beauty products and slimming aids to attain this state of 'perfection'.

All studies of the effects of dieting have shown that the most common outcome of dieting is a phase of bingeing with a rapid return to the original weight, or an even higher weight than when the diet was started. This may well be in part due to the problem described earlier – that when we eat less our body goes into 'fasting mode' and can become very efficient at eking out its supplies. This means that as soon as we start eating more again the extra is deposited as fat.

Glamorous comedienne Dawn French has worked hard to try to encourage larger women to feel comfortable and attractive just the way they are, and indeed her shop '1647' emphatically underlines the fact that 47 per cent of women in Britain in the 1990s are a size 16 or over! While it is laudable to help women feel better about themselves and to break the crazy cycle of dieting and bingeing that most people in the West permanently find themselves in, it is inescapable that obesity is linked with disease of all kinds. A healthy way of returning to a good weight is to combine better eating habits with the necessary emotional support and proper exercise.

THE ENVIRONMENT

The other vital reason we must change the way that we eat is the effect our eating habits are having on the environment. In the days when food was grown locally using low-energy technology, and eaten in the communities by which it was grown, the average input of energy was 1 kilojoule per 8 kilojoules of food energy being produced. Nowadays, because of the energy used in intensive farming – the running and making of machinery and fertilizers, transportation, processing, packaging and transportation of food to the shops (possibly right across the world), rehandling of the goods within shops, and transportation of the public to and from the shops to buy the food, there is now an input of 50 kilojoules of energy in food production for every kilojoule of food energy produced![7] This is an extremely dramatic statistic and makes it abundantly clear that we are on a collision course towards exhaustion of available energy resources.

However, most of what distorts this picture so greatly is the big shift towards the consumption of animal foods, which require so much more energy to produce than the production of plant foods. For example, it requires 10 times the energy input per pound of beef to produce the equivalent nutritional quantity of grain. In other words, we could feed 10 times as many people on a vegetarian diet than on a meat diet! The message is equally clear from the environment: we have to revert to eating a diet which is based upon vegetable rather than animal foods, which is grown organically and produced locally. Of course the most local place of all is our own garden, and this is the ideal solution – to start growing our own vegetables organically at home if we have any land whatsoever.

CANCER, DIET, AND THE IMMUNE AND REPAIR SYSTEMS

The important question for those with cancer and those wishing to prevent cancer is 'how does an unhealthy diet relate to getting cancer, and how can changing my diet prevent cancer or stabilize cancer once it occurs?'

The specific links with diet and cancer concern eating meat and animal fats, and too few vitamins, minerals and plant foods (which contain vital plant chemicals known as *phytochemicals*). Vegetarians are protected from cancer by the increased fibre, decreased fat, or increased consumption of a wide range of the phytochemicals present in plant foods found in their diet.

- Vegetarians are 40 per cent less likely to die from cancer.[8]

- The incidence of breast cancer is 30 per cent lower in those who do not consume animal fat.[9]

- The incidence of colon cancer is 25 per cent lower in those who do not consume animal fat.[10]

The non-specific factors include low energy levels, depletion in the body of important vitamins, minerals and essential fatty acids due to poor diet, and the poor functioning of tissues as a result of this and chronic toxicity. This, of course, is exacerbated by stress and the resulting poor absorption of food, as described earlier. As mentioned before, those who study disease in populations assess that 35 per cent of all cancer is caused by the Western diet;

another 30 per cent by smoking.[11] This means that 65 per cent of all cancer could be eradicated if we start taking a more responsible attitude towards our own health.

Broadly speaking, it would appear that it is substances in meat and fats which promote cancer, and the action of vitamins and minerals which protect us against these and other pollutants in our environment. A high-fibre diet helps by limiting absorption of cancer-producing factors; the active enzymes in raw plant foods also seem to convey protection and health. Vitamins and minerals also have direct stimulant effects on our immune system, and it is postulated that vitamins and minerals can stabilize and inhibit the growth of tumour cells directly.

All the repair and healing systems of the body are dependent upon good nutrition and a balanced diet, as everything from control of bleeding and the healing of wounds to the fighting of infection depends upon the correct balance of vitamins, minerals and adequate energy and protein back-up to take place effectively. In an overloaded toxic system, normal tissue function will be impaired – the function of the immune and repair systems included.

Another significant factor is that the body will attend first to stress or emergency situations. The excess of fat, salt, sugar or protein in the body constitutes a physiological emergency, and while this situation arises immune and repair functions will be compromised as the resources of the body go towards achieving homeostasis at the expense of immune function. A smaller but important factor is that when there is a great deal of extremely diverse material being fed into the body, particularly of tissue which is close in structure to our own, a great part of the immune system's function will be diverted towards recognizing these foreign tissues and making antibodies against them. Again, it is theorized that this may be a cause of some of the mystery illnesses of our time, as the antigenic stimulus from animal tissue may lead to the formation of antibodies to our own tissues, as occurs in the case of auto-immune diseases such as rheumatoid arthritis, thyroid disease and diabetes. Overactivity in terms of auto-antibody production and surveillance of 'invading proteins' from outside may distract the immune function from adequate surveillance of 'the enemy within' – that is, the formation of cancer cells.

However, it has already been mentioned that in a stressed, frightened, preoccupied individual the functioning of the immune and repair systems becomes secondary to responding to a threat in our environment, as a result of which most of us in the West have our immune function compromised already.

In the US there have been government guidelines since 1983 suggesting that to prevent cancer it is essential that we cut down our fat intake and increase our consumption of vegetables, fruit and fibre, and decrease our consumption of alcohol, food additives and smoked foods. In Britain, due to the pressure of the agriculture and food industries, and resistance from the medical profession, these guidelines have not been issued.

Recent study and research by the Bristol Cancer Help Centre has revealed the existence of 6,000 peer-reviewed scientific studies between 1980 and 1994 alone, pointing to the connection between the way we eat and our tendency to cancer. These studies have been collected on a nutrition database for study by those with an academic interest in this subject. The relationship between food, the way we eat and cancer could not be clearer from this mass of evidence, and for me the question 'Why change the way we eat?' has been answered definitively. To diminish the risk of cancer and all other diseases of civilization, and the abuse that our over-indulgent diet causes to our environment, we must all now rethink the way we eat as a matter of urgency.

Let us move on, then, to the question of how we go about it.

CHAPTER TWO

How to Change the Way You Eat

Some people, given the information about the need to change their way of eating, go away and achieve this in one fell swoop. I have known people who have returned from the Cancer Help Centre at Bristol, gone round their kitchen with a black bin bag, emptied into it half the contents of their fridges, freezers and cupboards and started into their new way of eating the very same day! I would have to say that this is a small minority, because for most of us changing the way we eat is very difficult due to lack of information about what to buy and how to go about preparing it. There are also time and money considerations, and emotional investment in our food and the way we eat (not to mention sabotage, however well meant, from our families and friends).

The most important thing is that the change is lasting and that you will not set yourself up for failure and stress, which would, of course, be entirely counter-productive to your overall state of wellbeing. It is therefore helpful if you are as well prepared as you can be before making the change, by anticipating your need for support, sufficient information, clarity and resolution about the exact approach you are going to follow, and specific advice about your own personal needs if you have medical problems affecting your eating, digestion, weight or excretion.

PREPARATION

The first key for achieving anything is to have sufficient support to do it! Usually the first place to start is by discussing the changes with your family. The ideal scenario is that your whole family change with you, as clearly this is an issue for everybody, not just those with cancer. Perhaps you could try getting them to read the first part of this book, or sit them down and explain how important it is to you and how much help you are going to need. If they cannot agree to join you, get them to agree at least not to sabotage you by offering you things which will make it difficult or, if you are the main cook, by expecting you to cook two different meals. Usually, if the family is old enough to object extremely strongly to changing their diet, they are old enough to have some input into the cooking of their own food; it would be wise to allow them to do so to avoid temptation *and* exhaustion! The availability of many vegetarian food substitutes which imitate meat products (such as veggie burgers, sausages, mince and stewing steak) make it very much easier to take a reluctant family along with you.

The next thing to do is to inform your friends and your place of work. This may feel quite intimidating at first, as you may fear that they will reject you or make life hard. Once you have got your new way of eating established, be prepared to ask friends over and show them how you eat by cooking for them. They will soon get the idea of what you need. It may also encourage them to take these steps themselves. Be prepared to take healthy food with you to work, and again sit back and watch how others begin to catch on to the idea.

You then need to decide on the level of professional support you are going to need. At the Cancer Help Centre there are extremely experienced nutritional therapists and cooks who can offer step-by-step guidance and support. You may feel the need to see a nutritional therapist regularly during the period of adjustment, and to attend wholefood cookery courses at the Centre or elsewhere. Do not deny yourself this level of support – it will make all the difference.

You may also have recognized, in the section on 'Comfort Eating' in Chapter 1, that changing the way you eat is going to bring up a lot of difficult feelings or make you feel very insecure. If this should happen it would be wise to see a counsellor. As your previously suppressed emotions arise, you will then have the opportunity of processing them and integrating them into the positive changes you are making for yourself. The benefits will then be doubled, as you will be tackling your physical and emotional state simultaneously. It is very important to take this seriously, because as with the dieting and bingeing cycle, unless the underlying emotions are sorted out your efforts to change may well be thwarted.

The other possibility if your partner or family will not support you is to find a 'buddy' or group who will do it with you. Perhaps persuade a friend, or team up with somebody you meet on a wholefood cookery course or at the Bristol Cancer Help Centre, so that you can discuss what is happening to you and thus celebrate and laugh about any triumphs and disasters along the way.

INFORMATION

The second key to success is to have all the relevant information at your fingertips. Hopefully by the time you have read this book you will feel this is the case, but again this can be a good reason to see a nutritional therapist regularly, so that your questions can be answered as you go along.

The information you will need is:

- clear dietary guidelines explaining what to eat and what not to eat
- a clear idea of what foods are available and what you should go out and buy
- an introductory meal plan to take you through the first few weeks
- nutritional information to ensure that what you are eating is balanced and healthy
- a good set of recipes.

All these areas will be explained in full in Chapter 3; a set of excellent recipes are available in the *Healing Foods Cookbook* by Jane Sen.

The third key to success is to be very clear about the choices you have, and your goals. By this I mean that once you have gathered and understood all the information about the healthy changes and what is available, you need to decide for yourself how far you are going to go, over what sort of period of time, and in what order. You may also wish to start the process with a 'spring-cleaning' diet (*see* Chapter 4), a fast or a period on juices, or alternatively you may wish to move into the process very slowly, making one small change at a time.

The entire process will be explained under the heading 'Planning' in Chapter 3.

The fourth important step is to talk to a holistic doctor (available at the Bristol Cancer Help Centre and via many natural health centres) if you have a cancer which is causing problems with eating, swallowing, digestion, absorption or excretion of food, or if you have weight problems. The doctor will guide you in modifying the dietary changes to ensure that you are getting adequate food, maintaining or putting on weight, and coping with any digestive problems.

The other major consideration here is chemotherapy and radiotherapy to the bowel. Chemotherapy causes slowing down of the bowel's activity and irritation of the lining of the bowel, which will create the need for soothing, relatively low-fibre foods during the time you are receiving this treatment. Radiation involving the bowel may also inhibit its function temporarily, and again care may be needed to adjust to a lower fibre diet. By and large, nearly everyone changing to a healthier diet says that their bowel function improves within a few weeks, including those with colostomy! However, it is wise if you have this or other problems to talk to the doctor first.

MAKING THE CHANGE EASIER

Ideally, changing the way you eat should be treated as a process of exploration and creativity – an adventure rather than a process of deprivation! The world of vegetables, fruits, cereals and pulses is an extremely rich one. There are thousands and thousands of wonderful vegetarian dishes from all over the world to experiment with. Do not forget – the majority of the world's population lives on a largely vegetarian diet, and people such as Madhur Jaffrey have opened up the world of Eastern and Middle Eastern vegetarian food to us, as have many other authors describing Mexican, Italian, Spanish, Chinese, Indonesian and French vegetarian cooking.

The other thing which I can promise categorically is that you will feel better once you start eating more healthily. Invariably those who make this step say they are brighter, more energetic and happier, and wake up more easily – not to mention all the other sorts of positive improvements in health, such as possibly clearing up allergies such as hay fever, asthma and rheumatoid arthritis. The skin becomes clearer and usually excess fat gradually drops away. It is important to know this, so as not to confuse it with the pathological weight loss associated with cancer. However, again it is better for those with severe cancer to have medical supervision to make sure all is going as it should and that excess weight loss is being avoided.

One way to avoid feeling that you are in a process of deprivation is to start by *adding* things to your diet before you start to take things away. The obvious place to start is by increasing your intake of fruit, making sure that you have a minimum of two pieces of fruit a day. Next, be sure that you are eating vegetables twice a day, and/or salad with most of your meals. Experiment with different ways of cooking vegetables so they become more and more interesting, and also with different types of salads so that these can become a bigger part of your way of eating.

The next thing to do is to start changing one meal at a time to comply with the dietary guidelines. Most people start with breakfast, as this is the easiest meal to change over, and go on to lunch and then dinner. Again, learn new skills before cutting away your old way of eating, and get to the stage where you know enough vegetable recipes to fill a whole week before you make the complete changeover. Establish a master shopping list of the things you are likely to need each week. Then use this as a master checklist before you go shopping (there is an example of one in Chapter 3).

Some people find that if they have five established main meal recipes which are quick and easy for weekdays, they can then use the weekend to experiment with new recipes.

During this process it is hoped that a subtler change will start to take place in your ability to care and nurture yourself with food. The holistic healing process involves becoming better and better acquainted with yourself and your needs. Learning how to feed yourself sensitively and properly becomes an absolutely concrete symbol of this more loving relationship with yourself, which you will then be able to introduce into more and more areas of your life. This does not only apply to feeding ourselves with good-quality, well-balanced nutrition, but also with the colours and textures of our foods and the rich creative process involved in thinking about it, shopping for it, making it and serving it.

BRINGING ATTENTION TO FOOD

Of course there is the question of how we eat our food. As discussed earlier it is clear that most of us need to set aside far more time for eating and digesting our food. I would strongly encourage you to return to the old rituals of setting the table and presenting food well, or creating your own rituals around food to enhance your enjoyment of it. Try not to rush away from the table as soon as possible – follow the example of our European neighbours who take an hour after meals at the table relaxing and enjoying the company of family and friends. If you are alone, perhaps you could try and relax or read a book rather than rushing off to do the next thing.

In these ways our food can begin to feed us on many levels – in terms of our creativity, our sensuality and our spirituality – and, like the Japanese tea ceremony, can become a form of meditation. You will find that the more focus, attention and love you give to preparing your food, the more wonderful it will taste and the more deeply it will feed you and heal you.

I once found myself in a macrobiotic restaurant in Rotterdam, Holland, called Zonnemaire. With each course that arrived I became more amazed at the quality of the food, but this was not only quality in Egon Ronay terms, but in the attention and love that had gone into preparing the meal. Each course was exquisite-ly presented, culminating in a plate of fruit salad which was made as a little miniature garden, with tiny branches of red currants standing as little trees among beautifully sculpted fruit and flow-ers. By the end of the meal I knew I was in the company of a very, very special chef. I asked to visit the kitchen and discovered that the chef was a Zen monk whose entire meditation was the grow-ing, preparing and serving of food. He allowed no chatting in his kitchen, and all his staff (who adored him) worked in a gentle, focused, loving and highly creative spirit. As he sent each meal up in the lift to the restaurant he personally blessed the food, and it was obviously his love, blessing and the attention he gave to the whole process which communicated itself in every mouthful.

Another outstanding example of this is the fact that, as already mentioned, a wholefood loaf has a 10-times bigger aura in Kirlian photography than a processed loaf – but an organic loaf which has been blessed has an aura twice as large again! We hear of the macrobiotic advice to chew each mouthful 50 times, giving full attention to the flavour and texture of the food while rendering it extremely digestible too. While this level of focus is not perhaps compatible with everyday living, we should aim to bring some of this quality of attention and consciousness into the way we prepare and eat our food, which will of course bring us into a far healthier relationship with ourselves, our food and our life process.

CHAPTER THREE
What to Change in the Way You Eat

The ideal diet for health, cancer prevention and treatment is a wholefood, organic, vegan diet which is supplemented with organic fish, poultry and eggs if necessary (due to excessive weight loss or very intensive medical treatment). The underlying change nutritionally that we should be seeking to make is to increase the amount of vegetables, fruits, cereals, pulses (and therefore fibre) we take in, and to decrease our intake of protein, fat, salt, sugar, chemical additives and stimulants. This will result in a cleaner, lighter, less challenging diet which provides optimum levels of nutrients and energy in forms with which the body can cope most easily.

The results of changing to this diet will be a rapid increase in energy, increased mental clarity, an improvement in skin and bowel functioning, and reduction in symptoms such as nausea, heartburn, constipation and piles. Changing the diet in this way may also have pronounced benefits for those with existing medical problems such as arthritis, asthma, eczema and diabetes, sometimes resulting in complete remission of these conditions.

Another vital benefit for those with cancer is that cancer treatment becomes far easier to tolerate. As chemotherapy and radiotherapy both produce toxicity within the body, if the body is dealing with a far smaller toxic load from the diet the toxicity of treatments can be coped with far more efficiently. Those who have had these treatments while first on an ordinary diet and then on a healthy diet have said that the level of nausea and debilitation they have suffered while being treated has diminished very significantly so ideally dietary changes should precede cancer treatment. How this translates into what we actually eat is as follows:

RECOMMENDED FOODS:

1   Wholefoods: All food should be eaten whole, with nothing added or taken away – e.g. wholemeal bread, brown rice, brown flour.
2   Fresh fruit and vegetables (not tinned or frozen) should be eaten with every meal, especially green, leafy vegetables – e.g. cabbage, broccoli, sprouts. Aim to have a minimum of five servings of fruit and vegetables each day.
3   Raw food – vegetables, fruit and raw cereals, nuts and seeds. Try to eat some daily as salads, fruit salads, muesli, or freshly prepared fruit juices – e.g. a mixture of carrot, apple and beetroot.
4   Organically grown food, as available and affordable.
5   High fibre – e.g. beans, pulses, lentils, vegetables and cereals.
6   Cold-pressed oils for dressings and cooking.
7   Variety: Avoid depending on any one food excessively.

FOODS TO INCREASE PROTEIN INTAKE IF REQUIRED:

1 Fish and poultry (and game) – deep sea fish is preferable, as is organically raised free-range poultry.
2 Eggs – organic free-range, maximum two per week.

AVOID AS MUCH AS POSSIBLE (ESPECIALLY IF INTENSIVELY FARMED):

1 Red meat – beef, pork, lamb, veal, bacon, kidneys, liver, salamis and meat pâtés.
2 Dairy produce – cheese, butter, cream, yoghurt and milk (use soya products instead).

Avoid Excess:

3 Sugar
4 Salt
5 Fat – particularly animal fats such as butter, and meat fats.
6 Protein – 2 oz or 40 gm per day is adequate, unless you experience sudden weight loss
7 Preservatives and additives, smoked or pickled foods – particularly barbecued foods
8 Caffeine – tea, coffee, chocolate, cola, alcohol, nicotine and non-prescribed drugs
9 Food which has been stored for long periods, irradiated, dried, processed, microwaved or repeatedly reheated

QUESTIONS ANSWERED

There are some questions which arise repeatedly regarding these guidelines. I have listed the most common ones here.

IS EATING BRAN A GOOD WAY TO INCREASE MY FIBRE INTAKE?

The answer to this is a categoric *No*. Pure bran is made up of fibre and almost nothing else and is highly irritant to the bowel. This is going from one extreme to the other; some studies have shown that bran is so irritant that it may actually be carcinogenic! It is quite sufficient to eat increased fibre as it occurs naturally in wholefoods such as cereals, muesli, vegetables, pulses and wholewheat flours and brown rice.

WHAT KIND OF FAT IS HEALTHY FOR THE BODY, AND IS MARGARINE REALLY BETTER THAN BUTTER?

The body does require fat in the diet – indeed there are substances called *essential fatty acids* (*see Glossary*) on which we are as dependent as vitamins for health. The best known sources of these essential fatty acids are fish oil, evening primrose oil and linseed oil, but in fact they are found in many seeds and nuts. The fats to avoid are the saturated fats found in animal foods, which will be particularly concentrated in butter, cheese, cream, milk, yoghurt and of course meat fat (unless you buy very low-fat versions of these foods and are meticulous about cutting the fat off the meat you eat). Even so, these foods are also very high in protein and daily intake usually pushes us into protein excess. The animal fats have been specifically linked to both cancer and heart disease. The recommendation, therefore, is to move to unsaturated fats such as vegetable oils, particularly cold-pressed olive oil for cooking purposes, and even then to keep consumption within reasonable limits to avoid excess weight gain.

The problem with butter and margarine is that many commercially produced margarines are highly processed and contain *hydrogenated* and trans fatty acids, which are also unhealthy for the body. These are produced by the processing and excessive heating of the fats in the production process. Because of this problem many people have given up and reverted to butter. However, there are margarines – such as Vitaquel and Granose – which do not contain hydrogenated fatty acids. These should be the preferred choice, as they are a good source of unsaturated fatty acids.

Essential fatty acids are not only vital for health, but have also been seen to have a specific role in cancer prevention and treatment. There are two families of essential fatty acids – the omega-6 fatty acids and the omega-3 fatty acids. The omega-6s are found in high concentrations in evening primrose oil, and the omega-3s in particularly high concentrations in linseed oil, fish oils and game. It is the omega-3s which have the most protective effect, and for this reason those with cancer are well advised to add a dessertspoon of organic cold-pressed linseed oil to their food three times a day for its protective effect (not the type of linseed oil used for the cricket bat, however, as this contains petrol!).

Originally the advice was to take linseed oil with sulphur-containing proteins such as those found in cottage cheese. However, subsequent studies have shown that it is as effectively absorbed with other foods, and can be added to soups, dressings or rice. Another way to take linseed oil is by grinding linseed yourself in a clean coffee grinder: 2 dessertspoons of seed provide about the equivalent of 1 dessertspoon of the oil, and again this should be taken three times daily sprinkled over food.

WHEN MIGHT I NEED TO SUPPLEMENT MY DIET WITH MEAT, FISH OR EGGS, AND IF SO, WHAT SORT OF MEAT, FISH OR EGGS SHOULD I BUY?

Contrary to popular belief (verging on brainwashing by a combination of our mothers and the milk and meat marketing boards) it is perfectly possible for us to exist on a vegan diet without fading away or becoming ill! Remember – great big animals like elephants, cows, whales and apes all survive on purely plant diets, which may encourage you to have more faith in the vegan approach!

However, those with cancer may have special requirements, either due to excessive weight loss or excessive tissue loss because of surgery or chemotherapy, or because they have a kind of cancer which produces a great deal of protein-containing fluid which has to be drained off, with consequent loss of protein from the body. In these instances it can become important to increase the protein intake with chicken, fish and eggs. It is always advisable to discuss this with an holistic doctor or nutritional therapist.

The other situation which creates a greater demand for protein is very intense physical activity where there is likely to be a demand by the body to build muscle tissue. This would apply to athletes, gymnasts and those involved in hard physical work. But even here it should be noted that Olympic long-distance runners are now using a low-protein/high-carbohydrate diet after witnessing the great success of the Chinese runners who follow this type of diet (only eating fish twice weekly)! Again, professional advice may be sought in order to achieve the correct balance in your own situation.

When buying meat, fish or eggs, the emphasis must be on buying organic. As already mentioned in Chapter 1, animals take in and concentrate in their tissues chemicals and growth-stimulating factors, and of course all animals raised with intensive farming techniques are likely to contain toxic chemical factors of one sort or another. Make the distinction when shopping between free-range and organic, because free-range eggs or meat may have been free to run around but may have been fed pure chemical food! When buying fish, go for wild fish rather than farmed or processed fish, as farmed fish will have been given chemically augmented food and may have been processed with dyes and flavourings. For example, much smoked haddock and salmon is artificially coloured and flavoured. The best fish is therefore deep sea fish and shellfish which have not been farmed. Deep sea fish include sole, plaice, cod, haddock, red mullet, bass, turbot, John Dorey and hake, all of which can form an excellent source of very high-quality, easily digestible, non-toxic protein. With shellfish take special care that these have grown in clean, unpolluted water a long way from a sewage outlet, as they are scavengers by nature!

Another idea is to go for wild game, but again be careful here because much game is reared by keepers to be hunted, and may also have been fed on chemically augmented food. If possible, check that it really is wild and not intensively reared.

The best source of genuinely organic eggs is to buy three or four hens and keep them yourself if at all possible, as they will supply ample eggs for an average family.

IF I GO VEGAN, DO I NEED EXTRA VITAMIN B_{12}?
Of particular concern is whether vegans get sufficient B_{12} to remain healthy – deficiency states can lead to anaemia. The answer to this is to ensure balance in your diet, particularly ensuring that you take in a good mixture of pulses, cereals, seeds and nuts every day, as well as a good cross-section of vegetables (including root vegetables as well as leafy vegetables and salads). If you are very concerned you can easily supplement your intake by occasional fish or B_{12} in tablet form.

WILL I LOSE WEIGHT ON THIS DIET?
It is very likely that changing to a healthy diet will cause the loss of excess weight, which will be very welcome for most of us. This is because of the decrease in consumption of fat, protein, sugar and refined carbohydrate.

The problem comes, however, if the diet becomes too biased towards vegetable, salad and juice consumption with insufficient intake of carbohydrates such as bread, pasta, biscuits and cakes, rice, cereals and pulses. There can be a tendency when first adopting this diet to this type of distortion, which ends up with you eating almost exactly what somebody else might eat on a reducing diet. This is because many people have read about anti-cancer diets made up of mainly raw vegetables, and have inadvertently lost the balance in their diet. The solution is simple. Make sure that balance is achieved (this will be clarified later in this chapter, under Planning and Shopping). The main rule of thumb, however, is that if weight loss has become excessive, build up the carbohydrate element of the diet by increasing your intake of pasta, rice, potatoes and wholefood biscuits and cakes.

WILL CUTTING SALT OUT OF MY DIET CAUSE PROBLEMS, AS SALT IS ESSENTIAL FOR LIFE?

Almost every foodstuff we eat contains salt, and without adding a single grain of salt to anything we cook or eat we will get adequate salt for our physiological requirements. The extensive use of salt in our cooking is solely to do with flavour and can really become quite addictive, with greater and greater amounts of salt being used. As with giving up sugar in tea or coffee, it is surprising how quickly we adjust and how quickly thereafter the taste of highly salted food is a real shock to the system.

One palpable benefit of reducing salt intake is a reduction of symptoms in those who have premenstrual syndrome and fluid retention. It would appear that the extra water retention experienced naturally towards the end of a menstrual cycle is exacerbated by the presence of a great deal of salt in the body, and that this can tip susceptible individuals into irritability, depression and all the other symptoms of this syndrome.

Some people try to achieve a salt flavour in their diet with the use of potassium chloride (*LO-Salt*) instead of sodium chloride. While this is less bad than sodium overload it still distorts the electrolyte balance within the body. It is far better to get used to the natural taste of foods if possible. Ways of bringing out the flavours in food will be discussed in more detail later on, and practical examples are given in the companion book to this one – the *Healing Foods Cookbook* by Jane Sen.

DO I NEED TO GIVE UP HONEY AS WELL AS SUGAR?

As explained in Chapter 1, it is important to wean ourselves off foods which contain large amounts of refined white sugar because of the stress which this puts on our system, the obesity it creates, and the satisfaction it gives without conferring nutritional benefits. High sugar levels in the body also predispose us to infections and have been postulated to create conditions in which cancer cells may thrive.

Having said this, glucose (which is a simple form of sugar) is the final endpoint for all our metabolic pathways and the source of all of our energy. As with salt, all of our foods contain sugars. Augmenting our natural sugar intake in a restrained way with the judicious use of small amounts of honey will therefore do no harm. Honey (unlike refined sugar) also contains other nutrient factors such as vitamins and minerals which are extremely beneficial to health. Overall, therefore, the careful use of honey is not banned if sweetening is required.

WHAT IF I CANNOT FIND OR AFFORD ORGANIC VEGETABLES OR FRUITS?

Try to go for fruit and vegetables which are as fresh as possible, locally grown and in season. Wash them very well and peel them if you know that sprays have been used. Buying local produce will at least mean that the foods are likely to have been left in the ground or on the tree until they were fully mature, as opposed to being ripened with gases on board ships in transport. It will also mean they will not have to have been covered in extra sprays for transportation purposes, or kept in cold storage for long periods with devitalizing effects on their enzymes. Again, if at all possible try growing what you can at home. Even if you can only manage a few rows of beetroot, turnip, lettuce or spinach this will improve the quality and flavour of your food no end, and give you immense satisfaction into the bargain.

DO I NEED TO GIVE UP ALCOHOL?

Ideally, yes. Alcohol is very toxic to our systems, most of all because of its intermediary metabolite acetaldehyde, which is what makes us feel so sick and weary. However, there are other factors within alcohol (particularly red wine) which are toxic and can give us nasty headaches and hangovers. There have been reports over the last 10 years that a glass of wine a day may help prevent arterial disease, but the evidence here is flimsy and it is quite likely that it is the relaxant effect of alcohol which is beneficial rather than any metabolic property *per se*. The whole thrust of the change in diet to prevent and treat cancer is to take the strain off the body, and so clearly drinking any more than one or two glasses of wine will begin to pull on the body's resources.

However, for many people alcohol is such a key part of their quality of life that to stop it altogether would constitute major deprivation. A good rule of thumb, then, is never to drink more alcohol than will give you even the slightest hangover, because the presence of a hangover means you have gone over into a toxic state. For most people this means that a glass or two of wine, or a pint of beer, is within the bounds. At the other extreme, however, is the occasional but severe 'not enough champagne syndrome' described by Cancer Help Centre founder Penny Brohn, which of course must be remedied immediately by at least half a bottle of champagne when we need rapid airlifting to our 'higher ground'!

DO I REALLY NEED TO GIVE UP
STIMULANTS SUCH AS CAFFEINE, TOBACCO
AND 'RECREATIONAL DRUGS'?

Almost every stimulant we use will put the body into a greater state of arousal. In these excited states we will burn up more energy which we may well need for our healing. As explained earlier, the state of arousal shifts the resources of the body away from the housekeeping functions into thinking-and-doing mode, which means that the maintenance work of healing and repair of tissues is compromised. Usually stimulants are used to help us escape how we are feeling. However, anything which causes us to go faster and bypass the normal signals of tiredness, hunger, sadness or depression means that we are failing to listen to the messages of our body and soul, and risk losing the integration and health of the system as a whole. It is far, far better to heed these messages – experience and express our emotions, and achieve our highs through the natural pleasures of love, communication, self-expression, creativity and sexuality.

However, as with unhealthy eating patterns, the habitual use of stimulants of any sort may well be masking an underlying emotional problem, and attempts to wean oneself off these substances usually requires having adequate support systems and counselling in place during the transition period.

It is comforting for those who love the experience of stimulants of one sort or another to know that all states which can be reached through stimulants can be reached through the practice of yoga, breathwork and meditation. If the body did not have the receptors to react with the external stimulants, then they would have no effect on us. The receptors are there because the body itself makes similar substances which can give us these experiences naturally;

an example of this is the discovery of the naturally occurring morphine within the brain called 'endorphin', which reacts with our own morphine receptors to relieve pain and give pleasure.

Through meditation, yoga and pranayama (breath work in yoga) altered states of consciousness can be reached, but when this is done naturally it is accompanied by an enormous sense of wellbeing, insight and self-love, as opposed to the chaos, danger, illegality and potential for overdose associated with the use of drugs and stimulants. Part of the danger is created because drugs produce mood/thought changes instantly in a body and mind which may be completely unprepared, and in social situations which may be completely inappropriate. The body's own 'stimulants' will be secreted in appropriate response to the situation or the amount of disciplined inner work and exploration one has made.

WHY SHOULD I AVOID FOOD ADDITIVES?

Many food additives cause no problem whatsoever, but there are others which have been found to be quite toxic, being implicated in cancer, behavioural disorders and allergy. The other problem is that many of them work by rendering the food inert and therefore less likely to rot. This compromises the vitality and nutritional benefit of the foods. In general, therefore, additives are best avoided if at all possible. This applies particularly to substances such as saltpetre (sodium nitrite) which is used for the curing of salami and meats, as this has been found to be carcinogenic. There is evidence from Japan that excessive intake of pickled foods has been implicated in cancer of the oesophagus. In this case, rather like the irritation of smoking to the lungs, it can be seen that very vinegary or spicy food may directly irritate the mucous membrane lining of the gullet and stomach, causing cancer to develop.

Another problem is in the smoking of foods or cooking of foods with barbecues. This applies particularly to smoking fish and meat, and barbecuing hamburgers, sausages and meats. It has been discovered that the hydrocarbons in the smoke disrupt the fat and protein structure in foods, creating carcinogenic free radicals which can initiate the creation of tumours in the body. One study on the subject suggested that if we eat barbecued food we should really precede and follow our meal with vitamin C, beta-carotene or vitamin E in order to deactivate the free radicals we have taken in![1] The subject of protecting ourselves with vitamins and minerals will be covered in Chapter 4.

HOW IMPORTANT IS THE QUALITY OF THE WATER THAT I DRINK, AND HOW MUCH SHOULD I DRINK A DAY?

Good, clean, fresh water is one of the most vital constituents of a healthy diet. Our bodies are composed of more than 80 per cent water, and it is in the passage of water through our systems that all of the balancing, cleansing and excretory processes occur. Natural spring water contains minerals which are essential to life; it is also well oxygenated, tastes good and feels alive to drink. By contrast a lot of our tap water tastes very chemical and may have an unpleasant 'used' whiff to it. Worse still, it may contain byproducts of the petrochemical, agricultural and plastics industries. Water filters within the house will partly clean up tap water, but do not by and large clear the chlorine or organic pollutants within the water. It is really a vexed question as we are so completely dependent on our drinking water, but water, like fat, is a universal solvent and readily takes up soluble chemicals.

The best solution would be to find a natural spring close to your home from which you could collect water regularly (having had it checked for cleanness by your local environmental health unit). The second best is to buy genuine spring water; it is a good idea to get advice from *Which?* reports and Friends of the Earth as to which brands constitute the best quality water available in the shops at any time.

The quality of our water is a matter of enormous importance and may yet be found to be a major factor in the increased cancer rates, particularly in hormonally-related cancers. In some reservoirs male fish have been rendered infertile by the presence of byproducts of the plastics industry which mimic oestrogen. It is up to all of us to lobby intensively for the cleaning up of our environment and water supply if we are to protect our health long term.

Once we have found a source of clean water, we should really be drinking around 2 litres (roughly 4 pints) per day. It is good to get ourselves back into the habit of drinking this as water rather than as squash, tea or coffee. This will be another good step in the process of detoxifying the body. Another idea is to try drinking water hot, especially in the mornings. This is helpful with elimination functions and as comforting as the first cup of tea of the day, once you get used to it.

HOW MUCH RAW FOOD SHOULD I INCLUDE IN MY DIET?

The use of food in cancer falls along a spectrum from food as therapy in its own right through to generalized healthy eating to support the body in all of its functions. Many of the cancer treatment diets which will be described in Chapter 4 of this book revolve around the use of a great deal of raw fruit and vegetables and of vegetable and fruit juices. If you wish to follow the generalized healthy eating guidelines, then the ideal is to have raw vegetables in the form of a salad with two meals per day, and raw fruit two to three times per day. The use of raw fruits and vegetables in juicing, 'spring cleaning' and fasting diets will be discussed in Chapter 4.

WHAT ARE THE BEST DRINKS TO FORM PART OF A HEALTHY APPROACH TO NUTRITION?

The most important drinks to avoid are those containing high levels of sugar, colourings and additives. Most 'pop' or fizzy drinks fall into this category. These should be replaced with either pure fruit and vegetable juices (preferably home-made) or the ever-increasing wonderful selection of carbonated fruit juice drinks which have been developed, such as *Appletise*, *Aqua Libra* and *Sao Rico*. If in doubt, consult the ingredients list on the bottle; do not buy any which have added sugars, colourings and/or flavourings. Gradually attempt to substitute tea and coffee with herbal teas and coffee substitutes. If you cannot give up tea and coffee altogether, choose the decaffeinated varieties for intermittent use.

COOKING GUIDELINES

As mentioned earlier there are some cooking methods which have been found to create carcinogens in our food. The worst offenders are barbecuing and smoking of foods (especially meat and meat fats), and the overheating of fat in deep-frying processes (and particularly the repeated use of cooking oils; this produces dangerous free radicals which can be potentially cancer-causing). It is therefore advisable to keep clear of barbecued meats and to restrict frying to a minimum. When you do fry, always use clean oil and do not heat it until it smokes. Many foods can be 'fried' in a little water, and cold oil can be added at the end for flavour and texture. This technique is often described by Kenneth Lo in many of his wok recipes using sesame oil.

The best cooking methods to master are steaming, stir-frying, stewing, roasting or baking food. Steaming and stir-frying mean that foods can be cooked quickly and lightly, thereby retaining much of their natural texture and nutrients. Baking, roasting and stewing foods are gentler ways of cooking which allow flavours to melt into one another on the stove or in the oven. The other technique to master is the making of a great variety of salads incorporating many different vegetables, fruits, nuts and seeds. It can be extremely helpful to invest in a good food processor, with shredding and grating attachments, for this purpose. In this way a coleslaw or mixed raw vegetable salad can be made in seconds. The food processor will also help in chopping and mixing nuts and other ingredients for nut roasts and vegetable pâtés.

Purchasing a juicer is also very helpful, not only for making up vegetable and fruit juices but also for preparing vegetable juice to use as a basis for delicious sauces which can be thickened with cornflour or arrowroot and served with main meals. Juices also provide an excellent and quick basis for soups. Juiced or puréed vegetables can also be used to replace oil in a vinaigrette. Jane Sen's *Healing Foods Cookbook* gives mouth-watering examples of all of these ideas!

For steaming purposes it can be helpful to invest in a small steaming unit which you can fit into any saucepan. These resemble flowers, with 'petals' that open. They stand on three small legs about one inch off the bottom of the pan, and are made of metal with many perforations. The 'petals' can open to varying degrees according to the size of the pan. The flavour of vegetables steamed in this way is a complete revelation for those of us brought up on boiled vegetables, and of course you do not lose all the vitamins and minerals into the water as you do when boiling them. There are a variety of other types of steamers available if you wish to steam larger quantities of food. The Chinese supermarket is often a very good source of different types of steamers as the Chinese steam much of their food.

Another purchase you can make at the Chinese supermarket (where they may well be cheaper than in an ordinary kitchen ware shop) is a good wok. This is a bit like a frying pan but has a gentle curved shape and (usually) a long wooden handle. This is ideal for stir-frying vegetables, as you can keep tossing the contents of the pan gently to make sure all the vegetables get cooked evenly. Electric woks are also available but are less versatile as it is not so easy to toss vegetables in them. It is also important to check that you have at least two good chopping boards (one for savoury and one for sweet), some good knives – some people like to chop their vegetables with a Chinese chopping knife, which is very fast and sharp. Basically you will need at least one good, strong, longish knife, a small vegetable and herb cutting knife, and a small mandolin-style vegetable peeler (which peels vegetables much more rapidly than the standard peeler). It is also helpful to have a pestle and mortar for crushing spices, and a garlic press. A real refinement is to have a clean coffee grinder for the grinding of seeds, nuts and spices for certain recipes, but this is by no means essential. While it is good to experiment fully with all the herbs and flavours available, it is wise not to get hooked on using too many strong spices, pickles or chillies, as these can irritate the gut lining and are thought in some cultures to promote the development of cancer in the gut. The other requirements – such as casserole dishes, pans, wooden spoons – form part of the equipment of any normal kitchen.

The safety of microwaving food poses a real dilemma. We are reassured that it is totally safe, but during microwaving very high-energy microwaves are put into the food, instantly causing rapid oscillation of the food molecules, and therefore very high heats. You will have noticed that if you try to eat something straight out of the microwave oven it is unnaturally hot in a very different way from food out of a conventional oven. We are supposed to leave microwaved food for a set 'stand time' after cooking in order to allow some of this very high energy to dissipate, but often we do not. This means that some of this high energy gets dispersed to the cells lining the gullet and stomach, which could have dangerous irritant effects.

There is also the consideration of what happens to the vitamins and enzymes within foods that are microwaved. We know they are destroyed by the high temperatures of frying and pressure cooking, and so again this does not bode well for foods heated so hot and so fast. There is also the more difficult consideration of what this blast of high energy does to the subtler energy or vital force of the food. So all in all it would appear safer to stick to traditional methods of cooking, or to use the microwave only minimally. At the very least, be extremely careful to follow the manufacturers' instructions about leaving food for the recommended 'stand times' before eating it.

In the main, you are trying to cook fruit and vegetables the minimum amount of time, to render them tender but retain their juices and nutrients. Flavours can be enhanced in a multitude of ways: with herbs, spices, vinegar, soy sauce, miso (a black bean paste), etc. – but I will leave the description of this to Jane Sen in her *Healing Foods Cookbook*.

FOOD REVIEW

Now is the moment to introduce you to the huge choice of foods you have at your disposal once you start to feed yourself in a healthy way.

Breakfast Cereals

The king of the breakfast cereals has to be muesli. Traditionally this is made from a mixture of four or five different flakes, such as wheat, barley, rye and oats, with a mixture of fruit such as raisins, sultanas and dates, and of nuts such as hazel nuts or cashews. Most healthfood shops now stock at least four or five mueslies which are augmented with other things such as coconut, apricots, sunflower seeds, pumpkin seeds, crystallized pineapple, dried apricots and figs. You have the choice either to buy one of these or to buy a basic muesli and augment it yourself with goodies to suit your own taste.

It is good to try to develop a taste for muesli with either soya milk, rice milk or fruit juice. It is particularly good if soaked in one of these overnight, as the dried fruit plumps up and becomes quite delicious. It is also good to cut fresh fruit such as apple, banana and/or grapes onto muesli for a really satisfying breakfast.

There is also a crunchier type of muesli which is called granola. This is made from cereals which have been coated with honey and toasted, and is quite delicious.

We have all heard of cornflakes, but it is also possible to get wheatflakes, riceflakes, buckwheat flakes, millet flakes and barley flakes. Some wheatflakes can be coated in malt or honey, and you can also experiment with puffed rice cereal and puffed wheat. In specialist wholefood shops you may find a delicious breakfast cereal called *Kashi*, which is a mixture of seven puffed whole grains and sesame.

Another lovely discovery is jumbo oats, which make a really satisfying porridge. They are bigger than ordinary porridge oats and have much more texture and flavour. They are also delicious in many dessert and biscuit recipes. Of course it is also fun to experiment with the traditional oatmeal porridges, and for this purpose it is quite wise to invest in a slow overnight porridge cooker, unless you have an Aga with a slow oven, and to buy good quality organic oatmeal. You can also experiment with other grains to make porridge, such as millet, brown rice, wheat flakes, rice flakes or even buckwheat.

Breakfast Fruits

A really lovely way to start the day is with a fruit compôte. Most dried fruits are sweet enough to make a beautiful syrup with the addition of water or fruit juice alone, and lightly stewed prunes, figs, apricots or a mixture of dried apples and pears make a really delicious start to the day. There is a wonderful dried apricot called the hunza apricot. It is particularly delicious if you stand it for 24 hours covered in water to which has been added a bayleaf and a few cardamom seeds. You then bring it to the boil and simmer it gently for 5 minutes only, then leave it to stand in the juice for another 24 hours. It is a really luxurious dessert, especially with a soya or nut cream.

The other thing to do with fruit is to have a lovely fresh fruit salad. This also makes a particularly satisfying breakfast. Alternatively, mix soaked dried fruit with the fresh fruit. As a substitute for yoghurt, try soya yoghurt and soya desserts. These are extremely good alternatives to their dairy counterparts and go very well with fruit compôtes, fruit salad or muesli.

Breads

Thankfully the age of bread has really come again, and most bakers, delicatessens and healthfood shops have a truly wonderful selection of wholefood breads. I recommend you try three-seed bread, which has a mixture of sunflower, sesame and poppy seeds; granary bread, which includes wholewheat grains; wholemeal bread or, better still, organic wholemeal. This tends to be less light than the bread we are used to, but is extremely tasty and packed with goodness. It is also possible to get a selection of Italian and Indian breads containing herbs, sundried tomatoes, olives and spices; these can add wonderful variety to your meals. Speciality bakers will also have breads made from rye, barley or rice flours as well as malted breads and fruited breads, which again make a delicious change. It is also possible to get wholewheat teacakes and hot-cross buns, which are good for breakfast as well as tea!

Fruit Spreads and Honey

There is an astounding selection of honeys available from good healthfood stores, from the delicately flavoured acacia honey to more robust, tangy buckwheat – from the creamy white clover honey to the dark Greek mountain honey, and the very sweet, translucent orange blossom honeys. Ideally you should get organic honey from bees which have not been sugar fed. You should use honey in moderation as on toast or in tea, and not in huge quantities as a pure sugar substitute.

As an alternative to honey there is malt syrup, rice syrup, corn and barley syrups, as well as pure malt extract. An interesting change is date syrup or molasses, each of which has its own very specific flavour, and of course there is maple syrup. This variety drives home the fact that so many foods contain natural sugars and it is fun to experiment with all the different flavours – again in moderation.

The area of fruit spreads is another joy to explore, and these can be used for preserves and cakes as well as on toast at breakfast. In most healthfood shops you can find a wonderful selection of sugar-free jams, including apricot, cherry, blackberry and apple, blackcurrant, strawberry and raspberry, as well as the more exotic varieties such as guava and mango conserve, banana and mango spread, pineapple and ginger spread, and peach and passion fruit spread! You will also find a dark, thick spread called pear and apple spread which is not the texture of ordinary jam but more like a dark paste. This is quite delicious, and the company who make it also make a pear and apricot spread. It is also possible to get low-sugar marmalade, and so toast and marmalade is definitely still on the menu!

Drinks

I have suggested trying to cut out tea and coffee because of their stimulant properties, but if you are unable to do this altogether then the tea to drink is called *Luaka*, which is a decaffeinated tea and a very pleasant one. It is also possible to get decaffeinated coffee both in instant form and as coffee beans. There are those who say that the process of decaffeination renders coffee more toxic than it is in its natural form, and that it may be better to have the occasional cup of 'whole' coffee than to have decaffeinated coffee regularly.

By and large it is better to develop a taste for herbal teas and tissanes, and again there is a startling variety. The traditional herbal teas are made from herbs, as the name suggests, the classic ones being camomile, peppermint, elderflower, hibiscus, lemon verbena, lime flower and fennel. However, the 1970s and 1980s saw an absolute burgeoning in the area of fruit teas, and you can get anything from lemon zinger, country peach passion, wild forest blackberry, Mediterranean citrus or mixed fruit and rosehip to pineapple and coconut or passion fruit vanilla! There are many other varieties too, and they are nice cold as well as hot. It is great in the summer to make up a big pot of herbal tea and then strain it and keep it in a jug in the fridge. The addition of some ice, fresh herbs (particularly mint) and a slice or two of fresh fruit makes an extremely refreshing and healthy alternative to cordials or sweetened drinks.

Another idea, if you are very fond of tea, is to move to a much more delicate type of tea such as jasmine or china tea, which can be drunk very weak without milk or perhaps with a slice of lemon. There is also the very distinctive and unusual Japanese twig or *bancha* tea, which is said to have anti-cancer properties.

This is made by boiling twigs and then sieving or straining the liquid to drink. It is quite delicious and brings with it shades of the Japanese tea ritual. Other unusual teas are *Mu* tea and *Rooibosch* tea; the latter is made from the African red bush and has a very distinctive, tangy tea flavour and far less tannin or stimulants. Of course with tea it is not just the caffeine we have to think about, but the bitter acidity of the tannin. If you try drinking your normal strength of tea without any milk in it you will be surprised at just how bitter it is, and many of us are subjecting our systems to this acid brew nine or more times a day!

There are many other healthy drinks which are sometimes used as coffee substitutes. However, I prefer to see them as drinks in their own right, not as coffee substitutes, as this does not create a false sense of expectation (none of them really tastes like coffee at all!). There is *Barleycup*, made from roasted barley, and *Yannoh* and *Bambu*, which are made from a mixture of grains, herbs and figs. There is also dandelion coffee made from roasted dandelion roots (which is a little more bitter), as well as the more chocolatey carob-based drinks which, if anything, resemble the taste of cocoa.

Juices

Juices come in all shapes and sizes, though those which are most commonly available in the supermarkets tend to be of a rather poor quality. This is because the juice is usually 'concentrated' (that is, most of the liquid evaporated off) in the country of origin, shipped in this concentrated form, and then diluted again for sale in the destination country. In this process many of the nutrients, particularly the vitamins and enzymes, have been damaged. Again it is better to get organic, whole, locally produced juice if you can. The best juice in Britain is, therefore, that made from apples, as we grow so many. A fresh organic apple juice will taste every bit as good as a fresh crunchy apple. Some supermarkets do sell freshly squeezed juices, however, particularly orange and grapefruit, and these are usually very good indeed.

Unfortunately many of the bottled vegetable juices have by law to be pasteurized. This is understandable because of the potential bacterial contamination from the earth, though again it is likely to affect the juice's nutrient content. The best solution is to buy your own juicer, scrub your organic vegetables clean, and make up mixtures of fruits and vegetables such as beetroot, carrot and apple to create your own absolutely delicious fresh juices. Of course when you first get your juicer most things in your kitchen will go into it as you experiment with everything from potatoes to turnips, celery and bananas! The bizarre thing with bananas is that they produce hardly any juice, though if you put a banana through the juicer and follow up with other fruits, the resulting juice will have a wonderful banana flavour. It is also possible to use the fibrous waste products from the juicing process to make a vegetable stockpot. In this way you will feel very virtuous as you squeeze the last scrap of goodness out of your organic vegetables! Again, remember to peel and discard the peels of non-organic vegetables and fruit before you put them in the juicer, as these can contain alarmingly high levels of pesticides and insecticides.

The New Drinks

Since people have cottoned on to the fact that taking in large amounts of sugar in canned drinks is such a bad idea for our teeth, metabolism, weight and nutrition, a whole new spectrum of drinks has evolved. These usually take the form of fruit juice concentrates diluted with sparkling mineral water. The first really successful brand was *Aqua Libra*, which has a very refreshing melon-like flavour; this was closely followed by elderflower drinks, apple drinks and other mixed fruit drinks.

There is also a selection of fruit juice concentrates available such as apple, pear, strawberry, blackcurrant and many more. Because these have all been heated in order to be concentrated, again they are not so good nutritionally but they do make wonderful natural flavourings for healthy desserts such as mousses and whips made with soya products. They can also be used to flavour the syrups in fruit salad, or to add interesting flavours to a sweet-and-sour sauce. Concentrates can also be used in place of sweeteners, because, being so concentrated, they are really quite sweet.

By far the best drink of all is good quality water. As mentioned earlier, if you can find a spring check the water quality and then regularly fetch yourself some fresh spring water, as it is absolutely the ideal water to drink. Failing this rather idyllic possibility, seek out the best quality bottled water you can find, and try to drink around 2 litres a day either cold or in herbal teas and tissanes.

Pulses

For most of us the image of pulses stops with red and green lentils, red kidney beans and dried peas! If this is the case for you, prepare to be very pleasantly surprised; this at first intimidating area of wholefood cookery will soon become a great delight. Pulses will become one of your main sources of protein if you choose to follow this diet, so it is important to work your way through any nervousness you have about cooking them so that you can really benefit from the wonderful variety of textures and flavours that are available. In the mean time, as you start to acquire these new skills you will be happy to know that many pulses are now available precooked in tins in the supermarket. While it is obviously better to cook beans fresh, there are occasions when convenience is most important.

Lentils

I did not mean to mock the red lentil – it is an extremely useful food which can be used to make delicious soups and Indian dahl, and forms the solid element in many roasts and bakes. Presently much more fashionable are the green puy lentils which have a delicious flavour and do not become as mushy as the red kind when cooked up. A nice alternative are ordinary brown or green lentils, and if you go into an Indian store you will find an incredible array of between 10 and 20 other types of lentils to experiment with. The Indian shopkeepers will happily tell you how to cook the different varieties; literally every time I have asked for advice I have been invited to the shopkeeper's home to be shown in person! The Indians, especially the Hindus, are usually wonderful vegetable cooks and they also have a stunningly generous attitude to food and its preparation. Following up on such an invitation can lead you into a real adventure, and may well end up in a long-term, highly educational friendship!

To make the most of the English lentils I recommend Rose Elliot's book *Not Just a Load of Old Lentils*, and for the cooking of Indian lentils or dahl I would refer you to Madhur Jaffrey's books, as her recipes seem to be foolproof!

Peas

The pea family is also quite large. As well as the dried green pea, which forms the basis of England's beloved 'mushy peas', there are chick peas (sometimes known as garbanzo beans), which can be used in stews, salads and also for the basis of the delicious Greek dish known as humus. This is made from chick peas, garlic, olive oil, lemon juice and tahini, and makes an extremely tasty dip or spread. There are also green and yellow split peas, most commonly found in soup recipes.

Beans

One of the finest and tastiest of gourmet bean is the flageolet. This is smaller than a red kidney bean, is light green in colour and has a delicate flavour. The other rather fine bean is the aduki bean, which is small and dark red and has a very rich flavour. Black kidney beans are rather like red kidney beans only a little smaller, and there is even another similar bean called a black turtle bean which comes from the US. These are both quite distinct from the small, very highly flavoured Chinese black bean, used to enrich sauces, fish and vegetable dishes and to make miso pastes for flavouring soups and stews. Black-eyed beans are different again: they are rather small white/tan beans with a little 'black eye' at one end where the bean adjoins the pod. Again, these are great for bean stews.

The large white butter bean is one of my favourites – it is wonderful to sauté cooked butter beans gently in olive oil, garlic and parsley, or to purée them as the basis for a dip or pâté. They also make wonderful soups and stews as they have such a rich, distinctive flavour. Cannellini beans are white and slightly smaller than red kidney beans, and form a very suitable main course bean. Field beans are round and brown and come from the UK, and take quite a lot of cooking. They are unusual and can add variety to your meal plans. Haricot beans are the ones used in tinned baked beans. In their natural state they are white; because they go such a lovely texture when they are cooked they are again ideal for soups and stews. Mung beans are small and green and are very often used for sprouting purposes, producing the bean sprouts so commonly available at Chinese restaurants. Pinto beans are rather pink and speckled, and again form a slightly unusual alternative.

The red kidney bean is most commonly known for its use in Mexican chilli dishes. Happily it is just as easy to make a chilli *sin carne* (without meat) as a chilli *con carne*; for most people starting out into vegan country this is a very easy recipe to master if you already know how to make chilli with minced beef. Some people keep, in fact, very close to the original recipe by substituting vegetarian mince products for minced beef (these will be described in detail later), but it is just as good to use beans alone. Red kidney beans also make a wonderful bean salad. Simply chop some onions, tomatoes, parsley and a little garlic, mix this with cold pre-cooked beans in a good vinaigrette and you have a lovely starter or main course salad.

This brings us to the most astounding bean of all: the soya bean. It is hardly ever cooked and served as a bean, but is instead the basis for a most astounding range of products. This includes soya milk, bean curd (or tofu), soya yoghurt and desserts, soya cream, soya cheese and many other soya pastes and pâtés, meat substitutes, and even soya ice cream! Babies can be reared extremely well on soya milk instead of cow's milk formula, and this is often the solution to lactose intolerance and the type of eczema/asthma associated with cow's milk and dairy foods. The soya bean is a small white bean which takes a lot of cooking to eat as a bean. To make milk it is simply ground and diluted with water. Like cow's milk this will then set to make yoghurt and bean curd, and the curd can be pressed just like cow's milk curd to make cheeses and more dense pâtés and pastes, which can be used in a variety of ways. Much of the vegetarian pre-prepared food sold in the supermarket is based upon soya.

Rice, Grains and Pasta

The starch component of our meals is the part which provides the main energy source, as starch is easily converted into glucose for fuelling our bodies. In the British diet the potato has long been the staple starchy food, while in most other parts of the world, especially Third World countries, the staple starch source comes from rice and grains. Rice and grains are far higher in vitamins and minerals than potatoes. They are particularly high in the B and E vitamins, essential fatty acids, vegetable protein and minerals (provided they have been grown in a good quality soil). In fact it has even been mooted that potatoes were introduced as the staple diet of peasants in the Middle Ages because it kept them less intelligent than if they were fed on a grain-based diet!

Many of the vitamins and minerals contained in potatoes and other root vegetables are concentrated 2 mm under their skins, and very often the skins are discarded. The same is true of rice and grains, and so it is important to go for whole grains – such as brown rice rather than white. Unpeeled scrubbed potatoes, boiled or cooked in their skins are delicious and very wholesome (if organic). In general, however, the aim is to eat at least one meal per day using rice and grains as the key element.

Rice

With rice the main choice you have is between the long-grain and short-grain brown rice, which comes from Italy, and the rather finer brown rice, which comes from Pakistan and is called Basmati rice.

Short-grain brown rice is not just for puddings (as is short-grain white rice), it just tends to have a slightly stickier quality when cooked than the lighter long-grain brown rice. This makes it a good choice for risottos, whereas I would recommend long-grain rice for a rice salad where it is more important that the grains remain separate and do not become at all stodgy.

For a real treat there is also a wonderful rice known as Wild Rice, which commonly comes from Surinam. This looks completely different, being much finer and longer than ordinary rice, and being encased in a black shell. During cooking the shells burst open and the rice swells, contrasting the white rice with the dark shell. The end result is very attractive, tasty and textured.

To cook most brown rices, one foolproof recipe is first to wash the rice and then add one-and-a-half mugs of water per mug of rice and simmer very gently until all the water is gone. Another method is to put a little bit of oil in the pan first, heat it, add the rice and stir it round in the oil, making sure all the grains get covered, then add the water, bring it to the boil and simmer. This method has the added advantage of flavouring the rice nicely with a hint of sesame or olive oil. Either method should leave you with a perfect result. No salt is added during cooking, and usually a lid is left on the pan at a tilt to allow for slow evaporation of the water. This usually takes 30–40 minutes. The end result usually tastes great just as it is, though you can also flavour it with olive oil, linseed oil, roasted sesame seeds or a little soy sauce. It may also be flavoured by the addition of either 2–3 bay leaves or 6–8 cardamom pods while cooking. Wild rice usually takes a little longer to cook; most packets of wild rice come with good instructions. Sometimes a little precooked wild rice can be cooked separately and mixed with ordinary brown rice to add a little glamour.

If you are planning to make a rice salad, it can be good to add your vinaigrette straight after cooking the rice, while the rice is cooling (having been drained of water), as this will keep the grains separate and the heat will help the flavour of the vinaigrette to be fully absorbed into the rice. Then, once the rice has cooled, it can be stored in the fridge in this way for later use, mixed with chopped vegetables, fruits, nuts and seeds. If you are intending to reheat the rice later to use in a savoury dish, then a small amount of olive oil only added while it is cooling will help the rice grains stay separate and reheat easily.

To expand your knowledge of rice cookery and your repertoire of delicious recipes I would strongly recommend that you study an Italian vegetarian cookery book to become familiar with the techniques used in cooking risottos, and Indian vegetarian cookery books for good recipes for pilau and biriani rice dishes.

You should also try rice milk as an alternative to soya milk. It is slightly less powdery tasting, and is therefore less likely to be noticed when used as a substitute for cow's milk.

Grains

If you are thinking that you are rapidly going to become bored with eating brown rice every day, do not worry: there is a wide selection of other grains to experiment with, some of which also have the advantage of cooking much more quickly than brown rice.

Wholemeal couscous is the first example which springs to mind. Couscous is made from wheat and only takes 20–30 minutes to cook. It can be used either as an accompaniment to vegetables or, like risotto, mixed with vegetables to make a main meal in its own right. Bulgar is also made from wheat, but has rather more texture and flavour than couscous. Both couscous and bulgar are used extensively in Middle Eastern dishes; many exciting recipes can be found in Madhur Jaffrey's *Eastern Vegetarian Cooking*.

Quite different again is the flavour and texture of buckwheat. Buckwheat has quite a strong flavour, which makes for an extremely interesting change. Its flavour is enhanced even more by pre-roasting the buckwheat prior to boiling it. In fact, all grains respond well to pre-roasting or toasting in a pan prior to boiling; you will find advice on how to do this in Jane Sen's *Healing Foods Cookbook*.

Another wonderful grain is pearl barley, which has a lovely texture and flavour and originates from the UK. We are perhaps most familiar with its use in soups, to thicken and enrich a winter vegetable broth, or perhaps in its other common use in the making of barley water. Traditionally barley water had lemon and sugar added to it and was often given to invalids as a restorative. In fact, on its own, without the lemon and sugar, barley water is quite alkaline and can be a great help in the natural treatment of cystitis. My main point here is that it can also be used very effectively as a grain in its own right as an alternative to rice, and again cooks more quickly than rice.

There are other whole grains which can be used exactly as they are, such as wheat, rye, oats and millet. The more you experiment with these different grains the more you will come to love their subtle and unique flavours and textures.

Another unusual grain is quinoa, which comes from Ecuador. This grain is particularly interesting as it contains all 22 essential amino acids – and is quite delicious. Finally, and highest on the list for entertainment value, is the grain made from maize – alias popcorn! Making your own popcorn is a riot and only requires a deep pan with a lid and a tiny bit of hot oil. You can render small children helpless with delight by putting far too much popcorn into the pan in one go, heating it up until it all starts to explode, calling them over to have a look, and then taking the lid off – which will end up with a fountain of popcorn shooting all over the kitchen, and your fun rating going up by at least 400 per cent.

Flours

Flours are made out of all the grains described above, and more things besides! Of course, where good organic, varied wholemeal flours come into their own is in the making of bread. It may be that, as with many people who have returned to this more natural balanced way of eating, that you get a strong urge to experiment with making your own bread. This has to be one of the most deeply satisfying forms of cooking, which brings with it a great sense of wellbeing and homeliness to all around you. It is a marvellous symbol of your intention to love and nurture yourself, and I recommend it whole-heartedly. It is wise to start with organic wholemeal flours, but if you progress and become more adventurous you could experiment with mixtures, including barley and rye flours.

There is also, of course, cornflour, which is ideal for thickening sauces, and gram flour (made from chickpeas), which is wonderful for making very light, crisp batters. It is often used in Indian cookery for this purpose. There are also brown rice flours, soya flour and even potato flour and buckwheat flour, which you will find in some recipes but probably not often enough to merit their storage in your kitchen.

Pasta

Pasta is another good way to get your starchy staple into a meal. Of course, strictly speaking it is a processed food and will therefore be slightly less nutritious than the grains in their whole form. None the less, for most of us it is a realistic and appealing way to cook and eat carbohydrates. As well as appearing in a multitude of forms it can also be made from the full spectrum of grains. Again, the golden rule is to go for brown rather than white pastas and to experiment with the different types of pasta to avoid becoming bored.

It is quite possible to get fusilli, lasagne, macaroni, penne, spaghetti, fettucini, tortellini, spirals, tagliatelle, shells and noodles in brown wheat pastas, and many of these different forms are also available in pastas made from buckwheat, corn and rice. Another interesting variation is pasta made from spelt, an Eastern European grain. It has a nutty flavour and is quite delicious.

Superior wheat pasta is made from the very hard durum wheat, which has a very high gluten content and an extremely good flavour. Nowadays it is also possible to get many pastas which are already enriched with herbs, garlic, vegetables, chilli and even soya. Where soya has been mixed in this will of course mean that you are getting your carbohydrates and proteins at the same time.

Pastas can be used in hundreds of different ways, with sauces, in salads, in bakes and as noodles in soups (most commonly found in Chinese cooking). The best advice here is to get hold of an Italian vegetarian cookery book. Once you tune in to the many different uses of fresh herbs, mushrooms, tomatoes, nuts and seeds, you will never look back! Nowadays there is also a wide range of extremely good vegan pre-cooked vegetable, tomato and mushroom pasta sauces for sale in supermarkets, which will be a great help for those with a busy lifestyle.

Nuts and Seeds

The use of nuts by the British seems to be confined to the purchasing of a large quantity for Christmas, which then lies around gathering dust until the summer (when they are finally, begrudgingly, thrown in the bin!), or the consumption of extremely salty peanuts in bars and pubs. Seeds, for their part, do not really feature in the average Western diet at all. In both cases this is really a great shame, because nuts and seeds form an invaluable source of protein, vitamins, minerals and essential fatty acids as well as being wonderfully varied in their flavours, textures and potential uses.

Nuts

The first thing to be aware of with nuts is the extraordinary difference between fresh nuts and nuts which have been hanging around for a long time in our shops and cupboards. Fresh nuts are usually soft and sweet with quite a creamy texture, whereas old nuts tend to become more brittle, bitter and increasingly rancid. Needless to say, then, it is important to try to get hold of nuts which are in season and as fresh as possible.

The most useful nuts in wholefood cooking are cashews, almonds, brazils, hazel nuts, walnuts, macadamia nuts and pecans. An absolutely delicious contribution from the nut and seed world can be made by the addition of pistachios and pine kernels to your cooking and salads. In fact both of these are so tasty that I would not be surprised if they never make it into the cooking pot at all!

Nuts can be used to form the basis of a roast or bake, which can be flavoured with curry spices, herbs or left plain for the natural flavours of the nuts to emerge fully. Nut roasts can be eaten hot or cold, and can be a wonderful substitute for the meat component of a meal. They can be accompanied by a sauce, perhaps made from tomatoes or vegetable juices, as the only criticism of a nut roast is that it can sometimes be rather dense and rich.

A little further along this spectrum, nuts can be used to make pâtés mixed with other ingredients, and of course puréed or processed in their own right to make savoury or sweet spreads. For example, hazel nuts, pecans, peanuts and almonds are all available as nut butters, whereas puréed cashew nuts, with the addition of a little soya milk and apple juice, make an absolutely wonderful cream topping for desserts.

Nuts, especially when fresh, can be curried with absolutely wonderful results. They can also be roasted either as they are or with a little soy sauce added to enhance their flavour, either to eat as they are or mix into salads, or for use as toppings on baked dishes. They can also be mixed into rice dishes, pasta dishes and vegetable stuffings. Whole chestnuts can become a delightful focus for a stew, or are absolutely brilliant puréed as the central ingredient in vegetable bakes and vegetable stuffings. Chestnut purée can also be used sweetened with fruit syrups as the basis for many wholefood desserts and cake fillings.

For tempting children onto nut butters it is possible to get those that are mixed with carob, which gives them a flavour similar to chocolate. Carob is used in preference to chocolate as it does not contain caffeine or other stimulants. Coconut is another extremely versatile nut. Like the chestnuts, creamed coconut can make a wonderful addition to a curry or vegetable bake, and serves equally well as a basis for desserts and cakes. Coconut also toasts beautifully in flakes for toppings which can be used on both savoury and sweet dishes. Coconut milk is, of course, also available, and equally versatile. Coconut cream is made from the puréed flesh of the coconut and can be used to great effect in drinks. For example, mixed with pineapple juice, crushed ice and fresh lime, you can create a wonderfully refreshing fruit cocktail; the addition of rum to this mixture creates the delicious *bahia* of the Far East. However, overall you should use coconut in moderation, as it contains saturated fats which have been linked with arterial disease.

Seeds

It is not really surprising that seeds should have such a high nutritional value. They contain within them all the essentials for the creation of a new plant. In fact the sprouting of seeds is another way in which their nutritional potential can be released and enhanced, as the sprouts become very rich in plant enzymes as well as the vitamins, minerals, proteins and essential fatty acids contained in the seeds themselves.

Seeds tend to be used either whole, plain or roasted, or ground into pastes or spreads. Many have such a high oil content that extraction of this oil becomes the main commercial use of these seeds. The most popular seeds for wholefood cookery are sunflower, sesame, linseed alfalfa and pumpkin seeds.

SUNFLOWER SEEDS

Sunflower seeds can be used whole in bakes, stuffings and top-pings, and are particularly delicious roasted in the oven after tossing lightly in shoyu or soy sauce. This way they can be used as a very good pre-dinner snack with drinks, or to go into children's lunch boxes.

SESAME SEEDS

Sesame seeds are tiny and extremely tasty. They are wonderful for adding texture and flavour to pastries, breads and savoury crumble toppings. Ground into a paste they form the delicious savoury spread known as tahini, which comes in light and dark forms. Tahini is used extensively in Middle Eastern cookery and is a very useful addition to vegetable stews (to add texture and flavour), as a side sauce with rice and vegetables, or quite simply on a piece of toast with margarine, topped for garlic lovers with a quarter of a clove of crushed garlic! It also forms the basis for the delicious Greek and Middle Eastern sweet called *halva* which will be described in the section on 'Snacks and Sweets'. They can also be roasted with a little sea salt and ground to form *gomasio*, which is described in the section on flavouring.

PUMPKIN SEEDS

Pumpkin seeds are large and oval-shaped with pointed ends, and are pretty tough-skinned. They are sometimes added to muesli and bakes, but personally I think that they are best left for parrots!

ALFALFA SEEDS

Alfalfa seeds are absolutely tiny and can be added to foods for their nutrient value, or used for sprouting the very fine, delicate sprouts which are now sometimes available in supermarkets and healthfood stores. This is a great relief for many of us who have ended up with rather smelly variations on a theme of our third-form biology class on the window sills of our kitchens – I certainly take my hat off to those who can effortlessly produce crunchy, delicious sprouts at home. No matter how you obtain them, alfalfa sprouts – along with the mung bean sprouts mentioned earlier – make a wonderful nutritious addition to salads and stir-fried vegetables.

The other seed you may well come across is the blue poppy seed, which has a fine flavour and a beautiful appearance and can be used in a variety of sweet and savoury dishes.

LINSEED

Linseed, as mentioned earlier, is becoming increasingly used as a supplemental source of Omega-3 fatty acids, and can easily be incorporated, ground, into many dishes.

Oils and Margarines

Oils

Oils can be produced from a wonderful variety of nuts and seeds. In the 1940s, 1950s and 1960s, along with the tendency to refine all other types of foods, oils were produced in such a refined state that it was hardly possible to distinguish the nut or seed of origin. Now, thankfully, there has been a return to natural cold-pressed virgin oils which retain both their natural flavouring and colouring. There is no comparison whatsoever between the delicious dark green virgin olive oil, dark brown walnut or hazel nut oils, or deep golden peanut oil with their insipid, pale yellow, refined counterparts. A small dash of pure sesame oil added at the end of a stir fry dish can add a wonderful depth of flavour, and the nut oils are excellent for flavouring vinaigrettes. Peanut oil is particularly good for Chinese cooking. Soya oil, sunflower oil, corn oil and safflower oil are less fully flavoured, but are cheap and wholesome. Almond, coconut and grape seed oil are rather more delicate and are sometimes used in cake recipes. Mustard oil, however, is not used in food at all, as it has a very high erucic acid content. Ghee, which is often found in Indian shops, is usually made from butter and as such is best avoided. However, some wholefood shops sell a vegetable form of ghee. In the main, olive oil substitutes well for ghee in Indian recipes.

Margarines

There is now a plethora of margarines available on the market, but actually very few of these are vegan. Most contain some form of milk solids and are best avoided (even many of the new olive-oil margarines contain milk solids). It is best to look carefully at the list of ingredients on the label. Two of the best vegan margarines sold in the UK are *Vitaquel* and *Granose*.

Soya Products

It has already been mentioned that the soya bean produces the most fantastic range of products, which is even more fortuitous considering that soy is now considered to be so beneficial. One of the first enormously helpful things for the vegan is the way that soya can be used to replace most dairy products. Soya milk tastes slightly chalky compared to cow's milk, but goes well with tea and on breakfast cereals. (It does not work, however, with coffee, as it seems to curdle.) Soya cream is remarkably good, and soya yoghurts – particularly if very highly flavoured with fresh fruit – are an excellent substitute. If you find it impossible to give up all yoghurt completely, goat's milk yoghurt is by far the best as it is low-fat and the proteins are very easily digestible. Sheep's yoghurt, however, is even creamier than most cow's yoghurt. For example, much of the creamy Greek yoghurt sold is made from sheep's milk. Soya cheese is perhaps the least good of the substitutes and may not really be worth including in your diet.

Soya beans are also fermented and made into an extremely good flavouring paste called *miso*, which makes an excellent replacement for the stock cube and will be described later (in the section on 'Spices and Flavourings').

The next stage along the soya path is into tofu territory. Tofu is a soft, rather jelly-like light curd made from soya milk left to stand and separate like curds and whey. The curd is pressed into square blocks which can be bought in brine from healthfood shops and Chinese supermarkets. This is what the Chinese call 'bean curd', and it can be used in a variety of ways. When it is incorporated into other dishes it is best to simmer it for a few minutes first to make it slightly more solid, otherwise it will crumble if stirred into sauces or vegetable dishes. It soaks up other flavours well, which is good because it is actually very mildly flavoured itself. Tofu can also be fried, which gives it a light brown, crispy coating. Skilled cooks can manage to stuff tofu with piquant sauces and vegetable mixtures and fry this complete to produce a mouth-watering snack or starter. There is a very light form of tofu called 'silken tofu', which can be used as a base for making quiches and cheesecake. Silken tofu can also be used as a base for vegan milkshakes and build-up drinks.

Tofu is also used mixed with other ingredients to form the base of many savoury wholefood products such as burgers, pâtés, pasty fillings and bakes. Apart from soya yoghurt, on the dessert front it is also possible to buy soya desserts called *Provamel*, which come in vanilla and carob flavours. These are rather like vanilla and chocolate custards, and are ideal desserts for children or as toppings on fruits and other puddings. Somehow they seem to be less chalky than most soya yoghurts, and children take to them very readily.

Meat Alternatives

There has been an extraordinary development in the past 20 years of a whole range of vegetarian meat substitutes, due to the burgeoning of vegetarianism. By and large these products are made out of textured vegetable protein (TVP) or Quorn, which is made from a myco-protein. This myco-protein, which has an extremely good nutritional profile (being very low in fat and very high in all the essential amino acids) was originally found growing underground in the Thames Valley and is now grown commercially in specially designed plants. TVP and Quorn can be made into a whole variety of meat substitutes because their texture is rather chewy, like that of meat. Quorn is slightly firmer than TVP, so a little closer to meat in texture. They do not naturally have a very strong flavour, but, like tofu, take on very well the flavours of sauces and marinades. TVP and Quorn can be bought as 'mince', 'chunks' (which represent stewing steak), or paste, which can be made up into sausages and burgers.

This is fantastically helpful for those who find that they wish to change over to a vegan or vegetarian diet without changing the type of meals that they eat. To help us even further there is now an increasingly good range of products on the market, with items such as meatless shepherd's pie, non-meat meat pies and vegan sausage rolls which would easily deceive the average meat-eater if only for the joyous fact that you never come across any offending bits of gristle or tubes! The only snag with this approach is that it may tend to keep you locked into the practice of basing your meals around large amounts of protein, but as long as you bear in mind the intention to reduce your protein intake to around 10–20 per cent of the meal, this is fine.

Biscuits

Happily, many savoury biscuits are already wholefood. For example, oatcakes are an absolutely ideal wholefood biscuit, as are many crispbreads. There are also the polystyrene-lookalike rice cakes, which are comprised of pieces of puffed rice stuck together. They are actually rather tasty, but the texture is one that some people love and others do not care for at all. They are especially useful if you suspect you may have a wheat or gluten allergy, and can be eaten with pâtés, spreads and jams.

By distinct contrast, most sweet biscuits are full of sugar and fat. You are far better off making your own, although you may find you have to be quite creative in order to bake good wholefood vegan biscuits. In general terms the best ones to go for are oat, fruit and nut based biscuits of the flapjack type, or wholemeal digestives. It is also possible to use stewed fruit purées and chopped nuts to make moister, more interesting and more delicious biscuits if you feel so inclined.

Dried Fruits

Dried fruits have been mentioned in the context of lovely things to have at breakfast time alongside your muesli, such as dried apricots, figs and prunes. Of course there are also dried peaches, pears, dates, raisins and sultanas. The undisputed king of the raisins is the very large lexia raisin, which is absolutely delicious. Lexia raisins can also be soaked and eaten as a fruit compôte, or mixed with other dried or fresh fruits in a fruit compôte.

The other types of dried fruit which are available are dried bananas, mangoes and pineapples. To my taste these are so far from the originals that I cannot really get too excited about them, but some people love them, either on their own as an alternative to sweets, or mixed in muesli and desserts.

The issue with dried fruits is the fact that, being so sticky and sweet, they are extremely susceptible to attack by moulds and bacteria in transit. As a result many of them are covered in sulphur, oils, insecticides and pesticides. Again, it is best to go organic if possible. You will tend to find that really organic dried fruit is dried more than treated fruit, so that it is less sticky and therefore less vulnerable to attack. This will mean that it is less succulent to eat raw, but will probably reconstitute just as well as the moister, treated fruit if left to soak. A good example of this is the hunza apricots already described, which, although sold in a rather tough dry nut-like state, soften after the two-day soaking process described (*see page 54*) into the most succulent delicious dessert imaginable.

It is rather nice to make your own jams and spreads by purée-ing stewed previously dried fruits; as mentioned before, these can form delicious bases or toppings for pies, tarts and desserts, especially if cooked with a touch of ginger, bay, cardamom, cinnamon or other spices of your choice.

Spices and Flavourings

There are far too many herbs and spices to discuss them individually, but again the best advice here is to try if you can to grow some herbs of your own, such as basil, coriander, mint and chives in the summer, and rosemary, sage and thyme all the year round.

Two other absolute cornerstones of most vegetarian cookery are garlic and root ginger. It is even possible to find or make ginger juice, which is like a ginger essence that can be added to recipes. It is also possible to grow or buy horseradish root, which has a very lively flavour grated into vegetables or sauces.

For most people the main problem is what to do about replacing salt. There is luckily a range of possible alternatives, including soy sauce, shoyu, tamari and miso: the first three are liquid and can be sprinkled over most dishes to add a salty flavour. Miso is a brown paste which needs to be mixed with water and then stirred into dishes to flavour them. It can also be used to make a soup or a savoury drink. These substances are still quite high in salt, but of course have other nutrients – particularly minerals – which make using them much better than using pure salt. Miso is often mixed with rice or barley and, coming primarily from the soya bean, is really a rich source of protein and other valuable nutrients.

Another helpful source of flavouring is in yeast extracts such as *Vecon*. These take the place of stock cubes, though again are rather high in salt so should be used judiciously. A teaspoon of *Vecon* with some boiling water can form a very pleasant savoury alternative to a cup of tea on a cold night!

The vinegar family is a very rich source of flavouring. Of course, in Britain we are the most familiar with the very harsh malt vinegars, but there are the much softer, more delicate cider and tarragon vinegars, and the absolutely delicious balsamic vinegar which is matured in oak caskets in Italy. This makes it much sweeter and more delicately flavoured than most vinegars, and absolutely ideal for most dressings and recipes requiring vinegar. For an interesting change it is also possible to get fruit vinegars such as raspberry vinegar; this, with a little walnut oil, can make a wonderful salad dressing.

While on the subject of salad dressings, I have mentioned already that it is advisable not to use too much oil. As a substitute it is possible to use fresh organic or silken tofu mixed with some onion, vinegar, mustard and a herb of your choice. However, I will leave Jane Sen to expand on this in her *Healing Foods Cookbook*.

Mustards and mustard seeds are a very good source of flavour and can be used in all sorts of recipes. Particularly good are the wholegrain mustards, or the fine French Dijon mustard, which can give a very nice piquant edge to a sauce.

Another idea is to use pre-made curry sauces, masalas, chutneys and pickles in your recipes. These can sometimes add a sweet/sour dimension to food, which can make it very interesting. Pre-made curry sauces, particularly the very authentic Indian ones found in Indian shops, can instantly transform a vegetable stew into a vegetable curry.

For the adventurous there is also the possibility of using seaweeds to flavour your cooking. These can be added to vegetables, rice or grains, with delicious results. The most commonly found seaweeds in healthfood shops are nori, combu, arame, wakame and hijiki. There is no way to describe the flavour of these seaweeds. Very broadly speaking the best results that I have achieved are by toasting the seaweeds lightly and then crumbling them and sprinkling them over rice, grains, bakes or casseroles.

If you find you are absolutely unable to give up salt, a way of cutting down greatly is to make *gomasio*. For this you grind toasted sesame seeds (that is, sesame seeds that have been roasted on a baking tray in a hot oven or tossed in a frying pan until they are deep brown) with a little sea salt (in a ratio of about 10 parts sesame seeds to 1 part sea salt). This is absolutely delicious and will convey a great deal of flavour without too high a salt content.

The other bit of good news is that it is still possible to include a little home-made mayonnaise in your diet. One egg yolk will hold about a quarter of a pint of olive oil beaten in drop by drop; to this you can add some balsamic vinegar or just lemon juice and, if you wish, some garlic. A small amount of this dropped into a bowl of tomato soup will enrich it beyond belief, adding tremendous texture and flavour, or of course it can be eaten with salads or on top of baked potatoes.

Another staple for most vegetarian cooks is the tomato in all its many forms. Perhaps most useful of all is tomato purée, which can be used to add flavour to many recipes. Another luxurious member of this family is the very fashionable sun-dried tomato, which is highly flavoured and can be used to bring all sorts of recipes alive. The same goes for the olive family. It is now possible to get all manner of good olives in Britain, but I think my favourite for flavour is the kalamata olive, which is firm, juicy and extremely tasty. Real lovers of olives will adore olive pâté, which is available in good healthfood stores and delicatessens and can be used in all sorts of ways to enrich food or to eat as it is on a cracker or with raw vegetables as a snack. It is also possible to get basil purée now, which means that it is possible to have the wonderful fresh basil taste even in the dead of winter.

Mushrooms are, of course, a subject in their own right. Many books have been written on the subject of mushroom cookery alone. I mention mushrooms here because often a very small amount can flavour an entire risotto or pasta dish. Special mushrooms include the French cepes, pleurotes or oyster mushrooms, bolets, and the Chinese shitake mushroom. Many of these are available dried; they reconstitute well when soaked and can then be sliced for use in stir-fries and other dishes: their flavour goes a very long way.

Cheese

'Vegetarian cheese' is a bit of a misnomer. What this usually means is that it is ordinary cheese made as usual from dairy produce, but without rennet in it. The reason for this is that vegetarians who do not eat meat on ethical grounds will not tolerate rennet, as it is extracted from the calf's stomach. It is an enzyme which helps convert the milk drunk by the calf into more solid cheese-like form of protein for digestive purposes. This makes it very useful for initiating the process of turning milk into cheese commercially. The only real vegetarian, or should I say vegan cheese is again made from soya – surprise, surprise! However, this is not really very like ordinary cheese and its use is somewhat analogous to using TVP 'mince' and 'steak'. In general, then, it is far better to get used to having genuine alternatives such as humus and vegetable pâtés rather than a pale imitation of the real thing!

Sheep's and goat's cheeses are more likely to be organic than cow's cheese, and goat's cheese has the lowest fat content of all three. However, they are still best avoided if you are to keep your diet low in animal fats and protein. Some cheese addicts attain high cheese flavour with low cheese intake by using a small grating of parmesan on their bakes rather than using any other type of cheese.

Snacks and Sweets

The most obvious area of wholefood snacks is nuts, which should be eaten unsalted and without dry-roasted additive coatings! There is also a large and ever-growing range of wholefood crisps and also tortilla chips – which, in their true form, are wholefood. However, it is worth checking the list of ingredients to make sure they do not contain chemical additives, colourings and flavourings. Popadums also make a nice snack and can be used for dips. Rice crackers, too, can be used for this purpose, but again look at the list of ingredients for the good ones.

On the sweet side, most wholefood sweets are based around nuts, dried fruit and seeds. Good examples are simply mixed fresh fruits and nuts, or nut bars, sesame snacks, dried fruit bars or halva, which is made from crushed sesame seeds and honey. There is, of course, also liquorice and liquorice sticks, which some people love to chew. It is advisable to get your children going on these kinds of sweets if at all possible before they acquire too great a taste for the extremely sugary sweets which are commonly available.

It is also possible to get or make pure fruit juice ice-lollies, which again are far better than the synthetically-flavoured and highly sweetened ones. They are also far superior to ice cream, which is packed full of animal fats and additives.

Baby Foods

It is actually surprisingly easy to get a wholefood vegetarian diet going for a baby. You will be pleased to hear that there is now a full range of organic baby foods available in the UK (the brand name is *Organix*). Good quality baby milks such as *Wysoy* are made from enriched soya milk. Many of the foods described already in the 'Breakfast Cereals' and 'Beans' sections will make very good purées for babies starting on solids, if mixed with vegetables or fruit purées and juices as appropriate. Soya yoghurts and desserts are also acceptable to most babies. The notion that babies love sugary things is inspired by our adult viewpoint: most babies will lap up healthy alternatives, and the wholefood habit will stick if started early enough.

There is an opinion that too much soya milk may not be good for babies, because it contains plant oestrogens. These can, theoretically, block the child's own oestrogen activity, which is related to sexual development. However, there is no evidence whatsoever that any child reared on soya milk has suffered ill-effects of this kind.

Fruits and Vegetables

There are far too many fruits and vegetables even to begin to enumerate them here. The key, as mentioned before, is to go with what is available locally and in season, with as great an emphasis as possible on buying food that's fresh and organic. Once you become confident with a few basic recipes, branch out and begin learning to bake and stuff vegetables such as marrows, aubergines and peppers. When you get more ambitious, try looking around Chinese and Indian supermarkets, where you will find more exciting challenges and flavours. Again, you will be helped greatly if you are armed with a copy of Madhur Jaffrey's *Indian Cookery* (not exclusively vegetarian but including many wonderful vegan recipes) or *Eastern Vegetarian Cooking*.

PLANNING AND SHOPPING

Now you have had a glimpse of the enormous variety which open to you, perhaps you are prepared to commit yourself to making the changeover straightaway. Perhaps, on the other hand, you feel that you are going to have to make the change gradually, in stages.

I will now describe a step-by-step process to help you decide exactly how far you want to go, how soon, and what help you will need. Just because you may not be able to take on board all the changes straightaway does not invalidate those you are ready to make.

Step One – Decision Time
The first step is for you to decide how far you are going to take it, and so I advise you to check down the following list and answer these questions for yourself:

1 Am I going to stop eating meat altogether? ☐
2 Am I going to stop eating chicken and game? ☐
3 Am I going to stop eating fish and shellfish? ☐
4 Am I going to stop consuming milk? ☐
5 Am I going to stop consuming butter? ☐
6 Am I going to stop consuming dairy yoghurt? ☐
7 Am I going to stop eating cheese? ☐
8 Am I going to stop eating cream? ☐

9   Am I going to stop drinking coffee? ☐
10 Am I going to stop drinking tea? ☐
11 Am I going to stop using salt? ☐
12 Am I going to stop using sugar? ☐
13 Am I going to stop eating refined and processed foods? ☐
14 Am I committed to decreasing my protein and fat intake? ☐
15 Am I committed to raising my intake of fruit, vegetables, cereals and pulses? ☐
16 Am I committed to drinking fresh spring or bottled water daily? ☐

Step Two – The Master Plan

I now suggest that you write your decisions out for yourself as a positive plan: in other words, for example in response to question 1 – 'I intend to stop eating red meat'; question 2 – 'I intend to stop eating chicken'; and so on down the list. This will really clarify and affirm your intention, and can be modified every few months as the change becomes easier and your intention becomes stronger. It may even help you to read your intention to yourself every few days, to strengthen your resolve.

Step Three – Support

The next step is to decide how much support you are going to need. First of all it would help to show your 'positive plan' of statements to your family or partner if you have one, and see if they are prepared to change with you. If not, explain to them how best they can support you and also how they can avoid sabotaging you, perhaps by suggesting they wait to cook their food until after you have cooked yours, or that they avoid buying things which are most likely to tempt you until you are well established in your new way of eating. Perhaps they could join you temporarily in your new way of eating while you get started, or could take on learning one or two recipes so that you can have a couple of nights per week off from having to prepare your own meals. Perhaps you can find somebody else – a friend, colleague, or someone you have met at a support group if you are ill – who will embark upon the new way of eating with you.

The next question is whether you feel that you are going to need a counsellor, nutritional therapist or doctor to see you regularly through this period of transition, especially if you know that you are compulsive about food, tend to use food as a sedative, or if you have a medical or treatment consideration which may affect the process. If you need help or advice in finding a suitable counsellor, nutritional therapist or holistic doctor, please do not hesitate to contact the information service at the Bristol Cancer Help Centre.

Step Four – The Game Plan

The next thing to do is to decide how you are going to tackle this. Many people find that it is easiest to change one meal at a time, perhaps starting first with breakfast and then going on to lunch and finally dinner. This may not suit you and you may instead choose to make the change in one go; again, make your intentions clear to those around you. It is also easier to start by adding healthy foods to your diet before you take away the unhealthy ones. For example, you could start by making sure you eat fruit several times a day, and have vegetables and a salad as part of your two main meals. You could then go 'wholefood' – cutting out refined foods, then gradually introducing more cereals, grains and pulses, and finally dropping meat, dairy produce, salt and sugar.

Step Five – Halfway There Already!

The next step is to identify as far as possible which foods, dishes and recipes you already know and like, and which fit into your master plan. Do not forget, for example, that simple things such as baked beans on toast, lentil soup, baked potatoes or porridge with honey fall into this category, as do most salads, fruit salads and many pasta dishes.

You may be quite surprised at how many things you already eat that are vegan, and how many of your usual recipes can easily be 'converted' with the use of meat substitutes. For example, it is possible to make a pasta bolognese, or for that matter a shepherd's pie, with TVP mince. It is also possible in the early days to have veggie burgers with brown rolls, relish and salad, so changing over to a healthier way of eating may not be quite as gruesome as you think!

Step Six – Meal Planning

I have already described an ideal wholefood breakfast comprised of muesli, cereals or porridge; stewed fruit or fresh fruit (possibly in a fruit salad) with soya yoghurt; wholewheat toast or fruit breads with margarine and low-sugar jams and honey, nut or seed spreads; accompanied by fruit juice or herb teas. Occasionally you may wish to have a cooked breakfast, with perhaps vegetarian sausages, mushrooms, grilled tomatoes and maybe an egg.

You will have to decide for yourself which will be your main meal of the day. As stated earlier, it is better to have the main meal at midday, but this may not be possible in the context of your working life. If this is the case, then the ideal lunch to aim for may well be a vegetable lentil or bean soup accompanied by either a salad made from salad vegetables, beans or rice. A possible alternative would be well-thought-out and delicious sandwiches, which could contain vegetarian pâté or humus with salad, olives or avocados. You may prefer a vegetable pie or pasty, or even a light pasta dish with salad. This can be followed with fresh fruit or freshly made fruit juice, or a soya dessert.

For your main meal you have many choices, starting with simple stir-fried vegetable dishes with rice or other grains, bean or lentil stews or casseroles, pasta dishes (including vegetarian lasagne), shepherd's pie, vegetarian curries or chilli, vegetable bakes or crumbles, pies, nut roasts, risottos and perhaps the occasional grilled fish dish with vegetables. Of course there are also all the convenience foods like Linda McCartney's non-meat pies, vegetarian sausages and so on.

You can probably cover yourself quite well for breakfast and lunches by shopping regularly for cereals, dried fruits, fruit spreads and basic vegetables from which to make soups, and a good variety of lunchtime salads. It is also possible now to buy very good 'home-made' vegetable soups in most supermarkets – for example the *Covent Garden* range of soups. Choose soups such as lentil or winter vegetable, however, which do not contain large amounts of cream and butter! To get yourself going for main meals it may then be advisable to write down a list of at least seven main meal dishes that you either know already or can learn to prepare before you make the change altogether. At the point at which you have mastered seven main meal recipes, you have probably acquired the minimum basic skills to make the change.

You may like to check which foods contain certain vitamins and minerals so that you can put extra thought into the planning of your meals. With this in mind, here is a table that should help:

A (Retinol & Beta Carotene)	Protects against infections, antioxidant & immune system booster, protects against many forms of cancer	carrots, watercress, cabbage, squash, sweet potato, melon, pumpkin, tomato, broccoli, apricots, papayas
B (Ergocalciferol)	Helps maintain strong and healthy bones by retaining calcium	herring, mackerel, salmon, other fish, dairy products, eggs
E (D-alpha tocopheral)	Antioxidant, protecting cells from damage, including cancer; helps body use oxygen, preventing blood clots, improves wound healing, good for the skin	unrefined vegetable oils, seeds, nuts, beans, peas, wheatgerm, wholegrains, fatty fish, tuna, mackerel, salmon, sweet potato
K (Phylloquinine)	Controls blood clotting	cauliflower, Brussels sprouts, lettuce, cabbage, beans, broccoli, peas, watercress, asparagus, potato, tomatoes, dairy products
C (Ascorbic acid)	Strengthens the immune system, fights infections, makes collagen (keeping bones, skin and joints firm and strong), antioxidant (detoxifying pollutants and protecting against cancer and heart disease), helps make anti-stress hormones and turn food into energy	peppers, watercress, cabbage, broccoli, cauliflower, strawberries, lemons, peas, melons, oranges, grapefruit, limes, tomatoes

B₁ (Thiamine)	Essential for energy production, brain function and digestion. Helps the body make use of protein	watercress, squash, courgettes, asparagus, mushrooms, peas, lettuce, peppers, cauliflower, cabbage, tomatoes, Brussels sprouts, beans
B₃ (Niacin)	Helps balance blood sugar and lower cholesterol levels, also involved in inflammation and digestion	mushrooms, tuna, salmon, asparagus, cabbage, mackerel, tomatoes, squash, courgettes, cauliflower and unrefined cereals
B₆ (Pyrodixine)	Essential for protein digestion and utilisation, brain function, hormone production; natural antidepressant and diuretic, helps control allergic reaction	watercress, cauliflower, cabbage, peppers, bananas, squash, broccoli, asparagus, lentils, Brussels sprouts, onions, seeds and nuts
B₁₂ (Cyanocobalamin)	Needed for using protein, helps blood carry oxygen, essential for nerves, detoxifies tobacco smoke and other toxins	fish, oysters, sardines, tuna, eggs, shrimps, cottage cheese, milk, cheese

Sample Menu Plan for a Week

Step Seven
The Shopping List: You will find life a great deal easier if you make yourself a basic shopping list which you stick to your kitchen wall and which you can check against each time you make your shopping list. When we have been cooking one way for a long time we have a mental checklist from which we make our shopping list, and of course this will now be different. You may also want to make yourself a 'don't buy' list, sticking it next to the other list to reinforce your good intentions. Increasingly there is a greater and greater amount of vegan foods available from major supermarkets, but I would still suggest that you take time to go and visit the best healthfood shops you can find in your area. If you have never been to one of these shops before, it will probably make quite an impact as you become aware of the large selection of foods available to you. This will contrast sharply with the experience of going around a supermarket and having the reverse experience, that is, having to seek out the healthy food from among hundreds and hundreds of items which do not fit into a healthy eating plan.

The following list can be used as a 'master list' to check against each week:

Organic wholemeal bread
Fruit bread
Savoury biscuits, crispbread, rice cakes or oat cakes
Wholefood digestive biscuits
Wholefood cake

Soya milk
Soya yoghurt
Provamel dessert
Organic eggs
Margarine (*Granose* or *Vitaquel*)
Oil (olive, peanut, speciality nut oils)

Tea – Luaka, herbal, fruit
Barleycup, Yannoh, Bambu
Mineral water
Fruit juice

Fruit spread (sugar-free)
Marmalade (sugar-free)
Honey
Tahini
Peanut butter
Humus
Vegetable pâté or spreads (such as *Tartex*)

Whole flours
Brown rice
Lentils
Beans

Cereals
Porridge oats (ordinary or jumbo)
Muesli (unsweetened natural muesli from healthfood shops)
Nuts

Seeds
Dried fruits

Pasta (dried or freshly prepared)
Noodles
Pasta sauces

Pickles (in moderation)
Mustard
Mayonnaise
Vinegar (including balsamic, fruit or cider vinegar)
Chilli sauce
Soy sauce
Chinese sauces (such as yellow bean paste, black bean paste)
Miso
Marigold low-salt bouillon powder
Black peppercorns
Herbs and spices
Garlic and ginger
Tomato purée
Chestnut purée
Coconut cream
Tinned tomatoes
Tinned red kidney beans or other pulses
Tinned sweetcorn

Vegetables – roots, greens
Salad
Fruit

Bean curd
Quorn – mince, chunks or 'sausage meat'
TVP sausages/bacon
TVP mince, chunks or 'sausage meat'
Fish
Pre-made soups
Pre-made pies, pasties and bakes

Books to Buy

To start with I suggest that you get yourself copies of:

Healing Foods Cookbook by Jane Sen (Thorsons)
Raw Energy Recipes by Lesley Kenton (Vermilion Press)
Indian Cookery by Madhur Jaffrey (BBC Books)
Eastern Vegetarian Cooking by Madhur Jaffrey (Jonathan Cape)
Ken Hom's Vegetarian Cookery by Ken Hom (BBC Books)
Leaves from Our Tuscan Kitchen by Janet Ross (Penguin)
Not Just a Load of Old Lentils by Rose Elliot (Thorsons)
The Bean Book by Rose Elliot (Thorsons)
Simply Vegan by Leah Leneman (Thorsons)
The Vegan Cookbook by Alan Wakeman (Faber & Faber)
Italian Vegetarian Cookery by Paola Gann (Optima)

The Indian book is not a vegetarian cookery book, and the two Italian books are not strictly vegan, though the latter do have many vegan recipes in them to give you inspiration. Nowadays if you look in the cookery section of any good bookshop you will find many vegetarian and vegan cookery books, and the BBC does a vegetarian cooking guide supplement each month.

IDEAL MEALS

I have mentioned again and again that we need to get away from the Western idea of basing our meals around a big hunk of protein. So what is the ideal meal?

Try thinking about the way the Chinese and Indians eat. Very small amounts of protein are cooked in sauces and then served with large amounts of rice, breads and vegetables. The idea is really to make sure that the major input in each meal is a mixture of carbohydrate and vegetables, or fruit. Roughly speaking, the carbohydrate element should form around 40 per cent of each meal, the vegetables around 40 per cent, protein around 10–15 per cent, and fat around 5 per cent. For example, some beans cooked in a tomato or vegetable sauce served on a bed of rice with a large side salad would be ideal. Alternatively, some stir-fried vegetables served with brown rice and braised tofu or stir-fried Quorn would be good. Pilau rice with nuts added to it, accompanied by a vegetable curry and dahl, also makes for an extremely well-balanced meal; or perhaps some soup and salad with humus and brown bread.

You will soon discover that by eating this way you will never feel bloated or nauseated after a meal, and that you will not experience peaks and troughs of energy in the same way as you do on refined foods. You will find that you have good quality enduring energy as the food is digested over a period of hours, and gradually you will feel stronger, healthier and far more alert.

TIMING OF MEALS

Try very hard to get into the habit of eating three meals a day, and if possible make your midday meal your main meal. Make time for your meals so that you can eat slowly and enjoy your food, and, particularly, leave adequate time for digestion after your meal. Try not to eat your evening meal much later than 7 p.m. so that you can allow time for digestion before you go to bed.

RAPID FOOD PREPARATION

The reason many people give for finding it difficult to become vegan or vegetarian is the time taken to prepare meals. I can assure you that once you are in the habit of eating in this way preparing meals will take you no longer than usual. However, there are tips which will help you.

First, it is very useful to keep some pre-cooked beans and rice in the fridge. When you cook either rice or beans, cook more than you need and coat the remainder with a tiny bit of olive oil. You can then use either the rice or beans to make a very quick salad, simply adding chopped apples, sweetcorn, red or green peppers, onions, etc. to the rice, or a little onion, garlic, parsley and tomato to the beans. With the addition of an oil and vinegar vinaigrette, you have a wonderful instant meal.

It is also possible to reheat the rice or beans for use in stews (beans) or fried-rice dishes. Simply make a sauce with onions, tomatoes, garlic, tomato purée and herbs, and add in the beans. In this way you can have a main course meal in the time it takes to cook your rice. Of course, tinned beans can be used in this way, too, as a convenience food. It is also possible to freeze rice and beans for re-use in these ways, or to make large quantities of bean stews, vegetable curries and pasta sauces and keep them in the freezer.

I must stress again, however, that the freezer should not be viewed as anything other than a long-term fridge, as the food quality will deteriorate. Aim to eat frozen food within three weeks of freezing it. If you can possibly make food fresh, it is by far the better course.

A food processor will vastly reduce the time involved in making vegetable salads, and if you keep a jar of vinaigrette in the fridge you can have a meal prepared in minutes. It is also possible to buy salad ready prepared from major supermarkets, although this is a rather expensive way of buying your salad.

Pasta meals can be ready within 10 to 15 minutes if you use a pre-made tomato sauce, for example. While the pasta is boiling you can make a salad, get the dressing out of the fridge and sprinkle some over it. It is also a good idea to make a big pot of soup once or twice a week. *Vecon*, which is a vegetable stock, can be used for extra flavouring, and quite a good tip is to purée half of the pot of soup in a food processor or blender and return this half to the pot, leaving the remaining thin cooking liquor as it is and the other vegetable pieces whole. This will give you a soup with a nice creamy texture and some bits of whole vegetable for texture. Sometimes if you purée the entire contents of the pot, the soup becomes far too thick and heavy.

The classic easy soups to master are lentil (made with red lentils, onions and tomatoes), leek and potato (vichyssoise), and onion. These three soups are very simple and absolutely delicious. If you take the time to prepare a lot of any one soup, you can have two or three meals stored in the refrigerator or freezer and ready to be reheated in minutes – and, of course, soups and stews improve if left to stand overnight.

SNACK ATTACKS

The second thing which floors many people's attempts to become vegetarian is the 'snack attack'. The things which people are used to reaching for are cheese and biscuits, sweet biscuits, cakes, crisps, salami, meat pâtés and chocolate. Part of this whole syndrome is the fact, as previously explained, that eating the wrong sort of food causes blood-sugar levels to swing between very high and very low, producing the tendency to want to snack or binge between meals. In this way we can easily end up taking in over twice as many calories as we need every day, and putting on far too much weight in the process, not to mention leaving ourselves feeling permanently exhausted.

However, we are never going to get away entirely from the need for snacks, and so it is better to be prepared with tempting, instantly available wholefood goodies, than to relapse into old habits.

The ideal foods for this are crispbreads and oatcakes with humus, vegetable pâté, yeast pâtés (for example *Tartex*), olive pâté and basil pâté. Having a good supply of first-class olives can also do the trick, or alternatively some delicious nuts or seeds. Ideally some pistachios, pine kernels, peanuts, cashews or macadamia nuts would be wonderful; tamari-toasted sunflower seeds are excellent too. Some people prefer a mixture of dried fruits and nuts, such as peanuts with raisins and sultanas. Dried fruit itself is excellent for snacking: the best candidates are dried figs, peaches and apricots.

There are many wholefood crisps or tortilla chips which are made purely from wheat and water, but do check that you are not buying products that are full of additives and salt. The other solution is to make yourself crudités out of raw vegetables such as peppers, celery or carrots, using these to dip into something like humus or a vegetable purée. The most important thing here is to think ahead and be prepared, so that you always have something in the fridge or cupboard when a snack attack strikes!

FAMILY TIPS

The ages of the people in your family will make an enormous difference to their willingness to accept the shift towards vegan food. Nowadays many teenagers are becoming vegetarians of their own accord, due to the extensive education in schools and on television about environmental issues. On the other hand, there are many teenagers who are extremely clear about their desire to eat meat, not to change their eating habits, and particularly not to do anything you (their parents) are doing. Usually if they are old enough to be this clear, they are probably old enough to have some input into their own cooking, and I strongly recommend that you let go somewhat of your role of provider and allow them to cook their own meals. Very young children, for their part, are usually quite amenable to things such as bean and vegetable purées and soya yoghurts and desserts. Somewhere in between these extremes, perhaps between the ages of 3 and 13, is the difficult patch. These children are usually extremely rigid in their eating patterns and highly influenced by peer pressure. With this group, the key is keeping everything looking and feeling as 'normal' as usual, and this is where things like TVP sausages, mince, steak chunks and vegetarian meat pies are worth their weight in gold.

It is always advisable to make changes as slowly and imperceptibly as possible, and to resist the urge to lecture your children about what's good for them – this will inevitably lead to stubborn resistance to all your efforts! Fortunately nowadays the media is more and more onto the healthy eating tack. However, often school catering is still in the dark ages; it may be worthwhile trying to get involved with influencing the meal policy in your children's school by doing a little lobbying via the school's parent-teacher group or board of governors. If your child takes a packed lunch to school, all the better.

VARIETY AND SEASON

While you will be ready to start your vegan lifestyle once you have mastered seven main dish recipes, your aim should be to go on experimenting and diversifying your range of meals. It is very important both nutritionally and for your own sense of creativity to continue to explore and try new things, as eating a good range of foods will ensure that you get a very good nutritional balance. It is also wise to change your eating patterns with the seasons and eat what is fresh at the different times of year. Foods which are fresh contain by far the most nutrients and vitality, and their flavour will also be best. The other distinct advantages about buying foods in season are that of course they will be far cheaper and you will not get bored.

Gradually, as you become more adventurous about experimenting with colours and flavours and new techniques, herbs, spices and foods from different cultures, you will realize that cooking in this way is infinitely exciting and satisfying, enabling you to feel happier and healthier than ever before, and really comfortable in your body.

STRESS AND 'FAILURE'

You are probably very well aware that the holistic approach to cancer and its prevention revolves first and foremost around reducing stress and increasing our happiness, fulfilment and pleasure.

It is very easy to see how changing the way we eat and giving up a lot of our favourite things can appear to be completely opposed to this underlying principle. There is also the definite risk that those who are very frightened by cancer can cling on to this dietary advice, becoming very rigid and obsessive and stressing themselves terribly if they lapse or are unable to maintain this healthy way of eating. It is extremely important to remember that the way we eat is only one part of the picture, and that the most important thing of all is that we are gentle with ourselves. Remember that if you are finding it hard this may mean that you are pushing yourself too fast, that you have insufficient support or information to make the change, or that there is another overriding factor, probably emotional or stress-related, which needs attention before you are going to be able to make the change completely.

However, as with all other areas of life, having the fundamental intention to move towards healthy eating patterns is the real foundation stone for the process. This will, for some, take weeks; for others it may take years. A wise friend of mine was asked about the process of creating intention: 'How can 10 minutes a day of visualizing the way I want things to be, possibly influence what I am thinking the other 23 hours and 50 minutes?' To this he replied, 'If a dog catches the whiff of something good on the wind and his nose turns towards where the good smell is coming from, then all the rest of him has to follow.' This is also true of good intentions: If you re-read your master plan to yourself every few weeks and reaffirm your choices to yourself, I assure you the changes will gradually take place.

The other thing to remember with nutrition is that it is what you eat the *majority* of the time that will make the difference, so the occasional lapse in your diet does not mean you have failed utterly. What you will find interesting, in fact, is that if you decide after you have been following the wholefoods diet after a while to have steak and chips followed by gateau and double cream one night, it will be very clear what this does to your body as it attempts to cope once more with the physiological stress of digesting large amounts of protein, fat and sugar! So the odd binge can actually have a very helpful effect in showing you the benefits of your new way of eating.

Seriously, though, be kind to yourself and do not 'beat yourself up' if you stray away from the path for a few days. Once you realize this has happened, perhaps get help or more support, maybe see a nutritional therapist again to get more encouragement, or repeat the process of making a master plan which is more realistic for your present needs and state. Trust that you will ultimately come out with the right diet which is perfect for your individual needs, by continuing to repeat this process every 2–3 months.

IDEAS FOR A WEEK'S MENU – BY JANE SEN

Once you are gaining in confidence you may like to try creating for yourself a week's menu from the following ideas:

Breakfast Ideas

1   Fresh fruit and/or vegetable juice
    Hot porridge made with soya milk and oats or brown rice
    (other grains are good, too: try cracked wheat or millet)
    served with dried fruits (prunes, apricots, figs, dates, raisins,
    apples, pears) soaked overnight in apple juice or water with
    or without some chopped mixed nuts

2   Fresh fruit and/or vegetable juice
    Granola-style cereal with soya milk and a sliced banana or
    two, or some fresh figs
    Slice of wholemeal bread, spread with *Vitam R* or *Vecon* and
    piled with thick sliced fresh tomato and a drizzle of olive oil,
    then popped under a hot grill for 5 minutes

3   Fruit salad of four or five mixed fresh fruits sprinkled with
    nuts (toasted coconut is lovely)
    Toast or rice-cakes with low-salt spreads, bean pâté or nut
    butter

4   Fresh fruit and/or vegetable juice
    Baked beans on wholemeal toast

Crispbread with unsweetened fruit spreads or honey
Fresh pear or apple

5   Soya dessert (e.g. *Provamel*) served with fresh fruit sauce
    (e.g. bananas, peaches, strawberries, apricots, raspberries,
    apples, pears, whizzed together in the blender or food
    processor), sprinkled with a little Granola-style cereal or
    toasted nuts and seeds
    Toasted muffins or fruit bread with soya margarine and
    unsweetened fruit spread

6   Fresh fruit and/or vegetable juice
    Compôte of dried fruits (apricots, dates, figs, pineapple,
    mango, prunes, berries, apples, raisins) either soaked
    overnight in apple juice or water, or cooked very gently until
    soft, eaten warm or cold. Serve with oat or rice milk, or, for
    extra luxury, nut cream and/or pancakes.

7   Fresh fruit and/or vegetable juice
    Organic cornflakes or cereal with soya milk
    Toasted wholemeal bread topped with slices of tofu, drizzled
    with tamari or tahini and popped under a hot grill with a
    halved tomato to brown
    Fresh fruits

8   Fresh fruit and/or vegetable juice, muesli with hot or cold
    soya milk (try soaking the muesli in the milk overnight to
    make it extra creamy and digestible)
    Toast or rice-cakes with a mashed banana and sprinkled with
    toasted sesame, poppy or sunflower seeds

The recipes for most of the following dishes can be found in *Healing Foods Cookbook* by Jane Sen:

Main Meals

1 Creamy leek and mushroom croustade
 Ginger and sesame carrots
 Lightly cooked green vegetable
 Tomato and cucumber salad with a parsley vinaigrette
 Fresh pears with almond 'cream' or soya dessert

2 Stir-fry of asparagus and brazil nuts
 Brown rice or noodles, with grated raw carrots and chopped
 spring onions stirred in before serving
 Shredded Chinese leaf, celery and bean sprouts with orange
 and sesame dressing
 Compôte of dried apricots (just cover with apple juice and
 simmer gently until soft), served with orange spice cream

3 Moroccan-style braised vegetables and beans
 Steamed couscous or bulgar
 Mixed green leaf salad with garlic vinaigrette
 Fresh strawberries and peaches, or apples and oranges served
 with banana 'cream'

4 Malay spiced tofu
 Braised sweet and sour carrots
 Rice or noodles with an equal volume of fine shredded
 watercress stirred in just before serving

Spinach and sunseed salad
Poached pears with fresh strawberry or raspberry coulis

5 Galette of parsnips and cashew nuts
Creamed fennel or potatoes
Lightly cooked green vegetables
Red cabbage salad with 'creamy' mustard dressing
Fresh fruit salad (made up of at least four different fruits)

6 Tagliatelle with 'creamy' mushroom and basil sauce
Mustard-grilled vegetables (aubergines, onions, tomatoes,
courgettes, etc.)
Mixed green leaf and cucumber salad with fresh tomato
dressing
Stuffed baked apples with blackberry sauce

7 Mixed vegetable curry
Spiced lentils of your choice
Rice or quinoa with shredded, steamed or raw spinach
Chopped tomatoes, cucumber and pink onions in 'creamy'
mint dressing
Juicy fresh pineapple

8 Braised squash with green lentils
Aromatic glazed turnips
Warm cauliflower salad
Fine shredded red and white cabbage salad
Italian almond pudding

Light Meals

1 Fresh sweetcorn chowder
   Hot granary bread
   Warm red cabbage salad with watercress and toasted pecans
   Two pieces of your favourite fruit

2 Poppy seed and sour 'cream' pasta
   Tomato, onion and olive salad with tiny leaf cress
   Fresh melon

3 Parsnip 'dabs' with sweet red pepper sauce
   Streamed or lightly cooked broccoli
   Mixed sprout and nut salad with lemon and cumin dressing
   Fresh pineapple and oranges

4 Grilled aubergine with *salsa verde*
   Middle Eastern rice salad
   Fresh peaches, plums or apricots

5 Courgette and potato rosti
   Broccoli, macadamia nut and garlic salad
   Fresh tomatoes
   Soya dessert

6 Quinoa pilaf
   Fresh tomato sauce
   Mixed green leaf salad
   'Creamy' avocado dressing
   Fresh grapes

7   Wholemeal bread or pitta bread stuffed with humus, Tunisian
    style carrot salad and shredded lettuce
    Slice of banana and hazelnut cake

8   'Creamy' cauliflower soup
    Spicy oven 'fries'
    Rosy red salad and chopped watercress
    Dried apricots, dates and figs

CHAPTER FOUR

Food as Therapy

I have mentioned already that the relationship between food and health can be seen along a spectrum, with healthy eating (which is relevant to everyone) at one end of the spectrum, and food used as medicine or therapy at the other.

When food is used as therapy, very specific, usually very rigid dietary regimes are advised with a view to perhaps detoxifying the body, dramatically raising one's energy levels, rectifying nutritional imbalances, correcting energetic imbalances, replacing deficient vitamins, minerals or other nutrients, or using a food, vitamin, mineral or nutrient as a medicine in its own right.

The other type of food therapy is the category of exclusion diets, where rather than adding foods to a diet items are withdrawn in order to see whether they are having an irritant or allergic effect on an individual's system.

Food is probably the very oldest form of medicine that we have. Human beings from every single culture on earth have realized the connections between what we eat, how we feel, whether we get sick and how we can be helped. This makes it all the more extraordinary that the role of nutritional medicine seems to have been virtually ignored by Western medicine in the 20th century.

The bottom line is that, as with any high-performance machine, the fuel which we put into our bodies has an absolutely direct effect on how well they work. Our bodies tell us in a variety of ways when the foods we are eating are not meeting our nutritional requirements, through the state of our skins, our hair, our nails, our energy levels, our gut's performance, nausea, irritability, irritable bowel, palpitations, allergic symptoms, and in many other ways.

There are two main problems, really – one is that very often those with a strong will or a determined or perhaps stoic spirit will chronically override signals from the body that all is not well. This, coupled with a great deal of ignorance among the medical profession as to the symptoms of nutritional imbalance and poor diet, and a tendency to treat these problems with drugs and procedures which often only make the situation worse, can often lead to the root of these problems going undiscovered, in some cases for a whole lifetime!

Apart from nutritional imbalance and deficiency, there is also the increasingly great problem of allergies, as foods become more complex, more processed and more changed by cooking and preservation processes. When this problem combines with the absorption of many other toxic chemicals from our environment as well as extreme stress and the long-term compromising of the workings of the digestive system, all sorts of problems and pathologies develop, including many of the auto-immune diseases, allergic conditions, cancer and arterial disease.

A good, well-qualified nutritional therapist is trained to understand the signs and signals which the body is giving us, and to tell you exactly where the deficiencies are in your diet, whether or not you are experiencing allergic symptoms, digestive problems or even infection with candida albicans (yeast) in the gut as a result of the way you are eating. He or she will also be able to give you the necessary support and information to alter your diet so that you can bring your system back into balance. This approach can be backed up by analyses of blood, sweat and hair samples, by firms such as Biolab, to measure the levels of minerals and vitamins in your system. In this way your progress can be monitored regularly. Blood and sweat analyses will give you a very up-to-the-minute picture of how your body is coping, whereas analysis of hair samples will give you a slightly more historical picture of what has or has not been being laid down over the preceding weeks.

It is also possible in some environmental units (for example, Dr Jean Munro's Brakespeare Hospital, near Watford) to have your levels of other chemical pollutants measured – e.g. heavy metals, petrol and petrochemical residues, insecticide and fertilizer byproducts, etc. It is actually possible to have blood 'cleaned' of these substances by the use of intravenous drips of vitamin C, and chelation therapy where these toxins are 'bound' to safe chemicals which are given intravenously and then excreted in the urine.

Chelation therapy can also be used to improve arteriosclerosis or narrowing of the arteries due to excessive fat intake and stress. Here the safe chemicals given intravenously combine with the fat inside the arteries, with the result that the arteries gradually become less rigid and occluded. This system is increasingly being used in preference to coronary artery or arterial grafting processes. Very often when grafting of arteries is done, the new arteries become occluded very quickly if the patient's diet is not changed at the same time, rendering this costly, frighteningly high-risk surgery virtually useless.

DETOXIFICATION

Many therapeutic dietary processes start with a detoxification, or 'spring cleaning', process. Using again the simple analogy of a machine, if you were to realize that you had been putting petrol in your car which was full of sludge and contaminants, the first thing you would go about doing would be to decoke or clean the engine.

The body has three ways of dealing with dietary excess and impurity: to metabolize it (break it down), excrete it, or deposit it in the tissues. When the excretory processes become overloaded, excess becomes deposited and our fat and body tissues become loaded up with chemical pollutants and partially digested meta-bolic byproducts.

The detoxification process usually revolves around stopping or minimizing input to the body for a period of between a day and six weeks at the extreme, in order to give the body an opportunity to complete the metabolic and excretion processes it would natu-rally be able to fulfil if it were not being continuously bombarded with more excess and impurity! For this reason some people make detoxification on a regular basis part of their way of life. The most famous of these was Coco Chanel, who ate only fruit and drank only pure spring water every Sunday, and who put her luminous beauty down to the regular observation of this cleans-ing practice. Of course, if we eat a well-balanced diet all the time it should not be necessary to detox on a regular basis, but quite often where there has been a long-term poor eating pattern, or where an illness seems to be related to the way in which a person has been eating, detoxification can be an attractive starting place to give the body the best chance of getting back into a state of equilibrium.

There are all sorts of detoxification and fasting regimes, varying from taking pure water alone to fruit juices alone, to having just fruit juices and fruit. Others go for brown rice fasting, feeling that it is less stressful to the body (since it provides a constant supply of carbohydrate energy and vitamins to the system). In the more rigorous methods where only water and fruit juice are taken, you are not only cleaning the body but you are also putting it into starvation, which has other medical implications and makes the body hang on to things rather than let them go.

In some regimes the use of coffee enemas is advocated to enhance the detoxification process, as this has been found to increase the liver's excretory functions several fold. It is certainly very noticeable that those using coffee enemas do become very bright-eyed and clear-skinned! This practice is much derided but is actually unanimously praised by those who have ever practised it.

Another very mechanical form of detoxification is the practice of colonic irrigation, where the bowel is flooded with tepid normal saline and literally washed out. There are many extraordinary tales of the startling material which can be passed as a result of this process, where the bowel has become impacted with the results of years of low-fibre eating. As with hardening of the arteries, this waste material sticks to the wall of the bowel and greatly inhibits its function.

A Cautionary Note

Fasting and detoxification is stressful and is a process which should ideally be undergone with medical supervision. Sometimes detoxification regimes provoke what is known as a 'healing crisis'. This happens when the input of toxins ceases. Toxins can flood out of the tissues back into the bloodstream and can temporarily create quite an unpleasant toxic state. This can temporarily exacerbate symptoms, sometimes quite dramatically, so it is ideal to have an experienced physician on hand to help you if necessary. Fasting is also inappropriate if you are already feeling very weak, toxic and vulnerable through illness or treatment. Unfortunately this is when detoxification is often embarked upon as a last-ditch measure. It is advisable that your condition be reasonably stable before you take this sort of step.

Simple Spring-Cleaning Diet

Having given all of these warnings, there is a middle path. Best known as a 'spring-cleaning diet', it entails putting yourself on a very clean, simple diet (comprised mainly of freshly made fruit juice, raw fruit, vegetables and salad, brown rice, cereals and lightly steamed vegetables) over a period of two to three months. In this way, without becoming hungry or having a strong detoxification crisis, you will very quickly clean out your system and feel very good indeed.

Cancer Detox Diets

There are many different sorts of detoxification diets, of which the most famous for those with cancer are the Gerson diet, the Breuss Juice fast, the Kelly regime, grape fasting, Dr Moerman's diet and Dr Alec Forbes' Bristol diet. In the Gerson diet a very high-quality organic vegan wholefood regime is combined with hourly freshly squeezed fruit and vegetable juices, and coffee enemas. As well as detoxification, the overall aim is to redress the body's sodium – potassium balance by providing a diet very low in sodium and high in potassium, with a view to restoring the natural vitality and 'electrical polarization' of cells. Recent evidence in favour of this theoretical approach has emerged, as the electrical polarization or 'transmembrane potential' of healthy cells has been found to be significantly higher than that of cancer cells. (*See Glossary for more about electrical polarization and transmembrane potential.*)

RAISING YOUR ENERGY LEVEL THROUGH RAW FOODS

All the old complementary medical systems and exercise forms, such as acupuncture, shiatsu, homoeopathy, yoga and t'ai chi, are based around the idea that we have a vital force or energy system which is strong and balanced in good health and depleted and imbalanced in poor health. One of the ways that our vital force becomes chronically undermined is through eating foods which are themselves very low in life-force due to intensive farming, storage, cooking and processing techniques. It is therefore obvious that filling the body with very fresh, live, raw foods can have a significant effect on raising energy levels and improving the functioning of our tissues. This rise in energy occurs because raw, fresh foods have the highest level of vitamins, enzymes and phytochemicals, which are normally denatured by heating and storage processes. This is the underlying philosophy behind the approaches of Lesley Kenton in her raw foods recipe books, and Ann Wigmore in her living foods diet and approaches where wheat grass is juiced and taken along with a predominantly raw diet (as in the Hippocrates diet).

All of these approaches revolve around making raw fruit and vegetables (either whole or juiced) a very large proportion of one's diet. Anyone who has ever tried this will tell you that within a very short amount of time they feel absolutely wonderful (provided that they were not too weak, ill or underweight before they started the process). Inevitably, eating this way will also cause fairly rapid weight-loss, so it is very important to find a sustainable balance which includes enough protein, carbohydrates and fats if you are going to stay on a very natural, predominantly raw, high-energy diet.

CORRECTING NUTRITIONAL IMBALANCES

While there are general nutritional rules and guidelines for healthy eating, it is never clearer than in the field of nutrition that each individual is unique. Foods and regimes that suit one person will not suit another. In fact, for some, dietary intolerance for certain foods and the resulting irritation to the bowel mucosa may be severe enough in their own right to start cancer. As described earlier there are many diseases and conditions which can have a strong nutritional component, so it is very important if you feel you may have a food-related disorder to seek the advice of a nutritional therapist. Of course, I have been saying throughout this book that cancer itself is a food-related disorder, but if in addition to this if you have an allergy or problems with digestion, malabsorption (imperfect or defective absorption of nutrients through the gut wall), pH balance (acidity/alkalinity) or candida albicans, your body's function may well be severely compromised. If you do have cancer, your body does not need to be labouring under any of these digestive conditions as well, and a nutritional therapist will be a great help to you.

Many people have found relief from chronic digestive, acidity and absorption problems by adopting variations on the theme of the Hay diet. In this diet the major focus is to eat either only proteins or only starches with your salad or vegetables at each meal. It is quite complex to follow, but there are excellent books around for guidance and it has certainly revolutionized wellbeing and made a very significant contribution to reducing the symptoms of diseases ranging from arthritis to angina!

Diets to help clear up candida (thrush) in the intestines are always aimed at reducing refined sugar intake, alcohol intake, and sometimes yeast intake. Sometimes the individual is also advised to take either caprilic acid or an antifungal preparation. This often undiagnosed condition can create a great deal of malaise, fatigue and cloudy-headedness, as well as abdominal bloating. Receiving treatment for this condition can be like turning on a light after a long period in darkness!

Another source of a whole range of diverse symptoms are allergies or sensitivities to certain foods and environmental toxins. Again it is very good to eliminate any foods to which you are allergic from your diet, so you are not depleting your energy or diverting the attention of your immune system to dealing with the offending allergen. And again, a nutritional therapist could help you to pinpoint those foods to which your body is sensitive.

CORRECTING ENERGETIC IMBALANCES

As well as the Eastern therapeutic and exercise systems which relate to the energy balance or imbalance of the body, there is also a dietary approach which works on this level, namely macrobiotics. In complementary medicine systems which look at the energy function of the body, the energy is seen as having positive and negative polarities, just as in electrical circuitry. In macrobiotics these two opposing qualities are known as *yin* and *yang*. The yin foods tend to be the sweeter, lighter foods, and the yang foods are heavier foods such as meat, eggs and cheese.

In a perfectly healthy individual, the aim would be to eat a diet where the yin and yang elements are completely balanced – so there are no 'forbidden' foods as such. However, to balance the eating of a 14-oz steak you would probably need to eat half a sack of brown rice! So once again we see that the basic guideline is to concentrate on the foods which are in the middle, between these two extremes, that is fruits, vegetables, soups, grains and cereals, in a ratio of:

grains and cereals 50–60 per cent
vegetables and fruits 25–30 per cent
protein as beans and soya products 5–10 per cent
soups 5 per cent.

This is extremely close to the current guidelines for healthy eating put forward by Western nutritional experts, in their understanding of the need for more fibre, fruits and vegetables without excessively high amounts of fat, protein, salt or sugar in the diet.

In somebody with a disease, however, the macrobiotic dietary therapist would be seeking to help correct the energy, or *chi*, imbalance by prescribing an individual macrobiotic diet, in which case the macrobiotic diet is definitely being used as a medicine or therapy. As with all these dietary approaches there have been notable successes – and notable failures – so it is necessary to have expert advice, clear information and very good support before embarking on this approach.

FOOD AS MEDICINE

The use of food as medicine comes under the broad heading of *Naturopathy*. Naturopathy is a very old, elegant and efficacious system of medicine. Many foods are known to have strong medicinal properties which can affect our mood states, heart rate and strength, digestive processes, liver functioning, tissue acidity and alkalinity, skin healing ability – in fact, every level of our functioning.

There are a whole number of foods and herbs which can be used to help with the symptoms accompanying cancer, such as nausea, pain, constipation and sleeplessness, but most exciting of all is the potential role of certain foods in the prevention and treatment of cancer. The most exciting work in the last decade has been done with green leafy vegetables and broccoli; yellow and orange vegetables such as yellow peppers and carrots; onions; and soya products. The cabbages and broccoli (and other brassicas) have been found to contain a compound called *indoleglycosinate*, which is anti-cancerous; the yellow/orange vegetables have been found to contain a combination of factors – including beta-carotene, calcium, selenium and micro-nutrients – which work in concert to produce a strong anti-cancer effect.

Soya products and fermented soya products such as miso have been found to contain phyto-oestrogens (plant oestrogens which block oestrogen activity, like the drug Tamoxifen), phytate, protease inhibitors, isoflavinoides and isoflavones, which are thought to be inhibitors of oncogenes – the part of the *DNA* in the cell and the chromosome in the cell nucleus which is thought to be responsible for setting off cancer cell proliferation. Studies with miso have shown definite cancer-protective effects. Lemons contain limonene, and tomatoes lycopene, which are also anti-cancer agents; shitake mushrooms, kombu and kelp also interfere with the *initiation* and *promotion* of cancer cells (*see Glossary*). Other plant or phytochemicals involved in cancer prevention under study are plant phenols, aromatic isothiocyanates, methylated flavones, coumarines, plant sterols, as well as naturally occurring plant selenium salts, ascorbic acid (vitamin C) with its accompanying bioflavinoids and co-factors (now thought to be as important as the vitamin itself), tocopherols, retinols, and carotenes. Many of these substances act in concert to render carcinogenic substances harmless, and to repair damage to DNA and RNA in the cell's nucleus, thereby preventing tumour formation.

The protease inhibitors like those found in soy are thought to protect cells from ionizing radiation, including the X-rays used in cancer therapy.

Dietary fibre also protects us in two ways: first through phytates and lignans, which directly lower the production of free radicals; and by speeding up the transit time of carcinogens through the bowel, thereby decreasing their absorption and harmful effects.

The criticism aimed at many dietary therapeutic approaches is that they can be very demanding in terms of time and money, and can lead to social isolation as well as to the tricky waters of the healing crisis (*see page 113*) and rapid weight loss. It is essential, therefore, that if these approaches are embarked upon it is done with adequate support, professional help and information. They are also often contradictory because of the differing underlying principles involved. The key here is to stick to one approach and not flit from one to another. However, with the emerging information about the specific factors within foods which may be protective, it may be possible to isolate the protective factors and incorporate the new findings into extremely specific and effective anti-cancer diets, thus avoiding some of the dogma and extremism of some of the dietary therapeutic approaches. It must be said that many people with cancer know that being positive and having a fighting spirit play a very important part in the recovery process, but it is impossible to be positive in a vacuum. Having an exacting dietary approach to follow can actually provide a framework for a self-help approach, and has for many people been an extremely important starting place, serving as a concrete symbol of their intention to do well and conquer the disease.

FOOD SUPPLEMENTATION – VITAMINS AND MINERALS

Frequently the response to the suggestion that vitamins, minerals and essential nutrients form an important part of cancer treatment and prevention is met with the comment, 'Why on earth do I need to take extra vitamins and minerals if I am going to be eating such a good diet?'

Certainly, eating well will exert a very large protective effect, but the issue here is that we are exposed to environmental pollution with petrochemicals, industrial byproducts in our water systems, farming residues of pesticides, insecticides, and the effects of ionizing radiation and increased UV light, and as such are potentially exposed to destabilizing chemical influences which can trigger the cancer process. Until we are in a position to make a significant improvement in levels of pollution, it is wise to take some antioxidant vitamin and mineral protection.

In general terms the reasons for taking extra vitamins and minerals for people with cancer are:

- replacement of long-term deficiencies due to Western eating patterns
- boosting of immune function
- deactivating of dangerous free radicals and pollutants
- direct stabilization of cell membranes and cancer cells
- possible oncogene regulation
- for those with cancer who may be facing rigorous treatment, to compensate for the tissue loss caused by surgery, chemotherapy and radiotherapy.

The relevance of the use of vitamins and minerals for those with cancer was taught to me by the Chief Medical Officer of Great Britain, Dr Kenneth Calman, when he was in charge of cancer services for the West of Scotland in 1985.

The Cancer Help Centre has created a database of studies on cancer. Between 1980 and 1995, there were over 6,000 high-quality scientific peer-reviewed studies providing a very solid body of evidence for the role of nutrition in cancer aetiology, treatment and prevention. As this database grows year by year, the number of studies per year continues to increase – yet most doctors remain largely unaware of this huge body of work.

The use of vitamins and minerals in cancer treatment protocols should now be routine, and all of us living in industrialized society would be well advised to take preventive vitamin and mineral supplementation.

> Vitamins beta-carotene, C, E and the mineral selenium given to 50,000 Chinese brought down cancer deaths overall by 13 per cent, and death from their most common cancers by 20 per cent.[1]

Some doctors feel that the doses of vitamins being given are very high, but these are based on levels which have been found in hundreds of trials to produce the best results. It must be remembered that most of the recommended daily amounts of these substances taught to doctors in medical schools are the amounts needed to prevent deficiency diseases such as rickets and scurvy. Clearly at this time we are looking at a very different set of demands on the human body due to the evolution and 'civilization' of society, which necessitates taking much higher levels of these substances. In fact, most mammals other than man have retained the ability to synthesize vitamin C themselves, and synthesize it at the sort of level that would be equivalent to our taking the recommended 3–6 gm per day.

Vitamins and minerals in adequate quantities are essential to health. They are needed by the immune system, and some may play a more direct part in protecting the body against cancer. Stress, illness and its treatment increase the body's need for supplements of this kind, and studies have shown that people with cancer can have relatively low levels of these essential substances. It makes sense, then, to ensure that the body is not allowed to develop a state of vitamin and mineral deficiency, particularly as many people also report that they cope better with radiotherapy and chemotherapy when they are taking supplements. This is backed by scientific studies.[2]

Retinoids (vitamin A) and beta-carotene (vitamin A precursor) have been shown to have very powerful anti-cancer effects, even returning cancer cells back towards normal in laboratory conditions.[3] Low vitamin A levels are linked with cancer of the colon, lung, cervix, larynx, bladder, oesophagus, stomach, rectum, prostate and mouth.[4] However, paradoxically, recent studies have shown that smokers who take beta-carotene may be at *increased* risk of cancer. Obviously I would suggest giving up the cigarettes rather than the beta-carotene![5]

Hundreds of vitamin C studies have shown a preventive effect of vitamin C on cancer.[6] Vitamin C is the fastest free radical scavenger and can also improve our oxygen supply by improving the blood's haemoglobin status. Its effectiveness can be enhanced by vitamin K and chelated iron.

Stress lowers our vitamin C levels, which is yet another reason why stress leaves us so vulnerable. Low vitamin C levels have been found in people with cancer of the uterus, cervix and ovary, and in those with leukaemia and lymphoma.[7]

Vitamin E is also antioxidant, and also potentiates selenium, especially in the natural tocopherol form (rather than as the synthetic succinate). Selenium is itself a preventive or resistance factor in cancer, as it protects against free radicals, mutagens, toxic heavy metals and certain bacterial, viral and fungal pathogens.[8]

The Bristol Cancer Help Centre
Vitamin and Mineral Supplementation Regime –
Recommended Dosages:

During Active Phases of Cancer

Vitamin C (as calcium or magnesium ascorbate)	Start with 500 mg 3 times daily, and increase gradually to 2 grammes 3 times daily

Please note: If you get an upset stomach, reduce the dose and stick to the level which does not cause diarrhoea. The ascorbic acid form is best avoided as this can be too acidic, causing stomach upsets at lower levels.

Beta-carotene	15 mg capsule once daily, or 3 x 6-mg tablets once daily (approximately 30,000 iu daily). Half a pint of carrot juice is equivalent to 6 mg or 10,000 iu, so reduce tablet dose accordingly if taking juice. Beta-carotene is the safe form in which to take vitamin A.

Please note: This is a pigment and may occasionally cause the skin to turn orange. If this happens, reduce dose but do not worry. The staining of the skin will not harm you, and will soon fade as levels drop.

Selenium	200 micrograms daily
Vitamin E	400 iu daily

Please note: There is some controversy over the use of vitamins in hormone-dependent cancers (that is, breast, uterus, ovarian, prostate and testicular), as it may boost hormone levels. The Bristol Cancer Help Centre therefore recommends that vitamin E is omitted by sufferers of these forms of cancer.

Vitamin B complex – optional	50 mg daily. B complex contains most of the B vitamins in one tablet.

Please note: this may turn your urine bright yellow, but there is no need to be concerned about this.

Zinc orotate (or gluconate)	100 mg daily, or Zinc citrate 50 mg daily.

This provides 15 mg of elemental zinc. Zinc is not well absorbed, so it is best not taken with food; this can easily be achieved by taking it last thing at night. It is gradually accumulated in the body, so reduce the dose to 30 mg zinc orotate (15 mg zinc citrate) daily (approximately 5 mg elemental zinc) after about three months. Resume at the higher level for a further three months if you have a recurrence or further treatment.

When You Are In Remission

Continue with:

Vitamin C	1 gm 3 times daily
Beta-carotene	12–15 mg daily
Selenium	200 micrograms daily
Vitamin E	200 iu (see vitamin E note above, regarding hormone-dependent cancers)
Zinc orotate	30 mg daily (elemental zinc 5 mg daily)
Vitamin B complex	50 mg daily

Vitamins and Minerals During Radiotherapy and Chemotherapy

Vitamin C augments the effectiveness of radiotherapy and can help decrease the anaemia, pain, appetite loss and weight loss experienced by those on this form of treatment. Vitamin C also protects the heart for those on the chemotherapeutic drug Adriamycin (as does co-enzyme Q10 or Ubiquinone).[9] Vitamin C also enhances the effectiveness of chemotherapeutic agents 5-Fluo-uracil and Bleomycin. Vitamin E reduces cardiac and skin toxicity and hair loss for those on Doxorubicin, protects lymph tissue against Bleomycin, and decreases cardio-toxicity of Adriamycin. Beta-carotene potentiates the effectiveness of 5-Fluo-uracil, Methotrexate and Cobalt therapy. Selenium is also radio- and chemo-protective, and protects the kidneys against cisplatin. Radiotherapy decreases levels of vitamin E, B_{12}, folic acid and C, so it is a good idea to ensure either a diet rich in these substances or supplementation while on radiotherapy.[10]

Remedies During Chemotherapy

For abdominal disturbances, take Aloe Vera Juice (1 dsp 3 times a day); or slippery elm powder (1 tsp 3 times a day) in a concentrated herb tea or mixed with soya milk or yoghurt; or comfrey tea (3 times per day).

FOR NAUSEA

Try root ginger, grated or as a tea (also available as tea-bags). Some people also find sea-bands useful: these are bands worn on the wrist and are marketed for use against sea-sickness. They work by exerting pressure on relevant acupuncture points through little pads, and are remarkably effective. Most chemists stock them. Slippery elm is also often useful for nausea.

Radiotherapy

The side-effects of radiotherapy may be helped by Homoeopathic Radiation Remedy (obtainable from Galen Homoeopathics, Lewell Mill, West Stafford, near Dorchester). Aloe Vera and vitamin E cream or Louise Brackenbury's Aromatherapy Radiation Cream (obtainable from the shop at Bristol Cancer Help Centre) may be used to protect your skin during and after radiotherapy.

PROBLEMS SWALLOWING PILLS AND CAPSULES

Many vitamins can be obtained in droplet form. Most tablets can be crushed and capsules pierced to make them palatable by mixing them in fruit juice or soup.

PROBLEMS WITH ABSORPTION

If you suspect, for whatever reason, that you may have a problem absorbing vitamins, you might consider using sub-lingual products, designed to be absorbed under the tongue or in the cheek cavity.

Cancer Prevention

With growing evidence that cancer may be prevented by adequate levels of antioxidants, the following regime can be recommended:

Vitamin C as calcium or magnesium ascorbate	500 mg 3 times per day
Beta-carotene	12 to 15 mg, once per day
Vitamin E	200 iu, once per day
Selenium	200 micrograms, once per day
Vitamin B complex	50 mg strength, once per day

COENZYME Q10 OR UBIQUINONE

This substance is receiving a great deal of attention as a potential protection and treatment in cancer. It forms part of the energy-producing mechanism in cells, and has an antioxidant function. In a Danish study of women with breast cancer, many women experienced pronounced improvement of their condition. In the study, the women took up to 300 mg per day.[11] For prevention purposes, 90 mg per day would seem to be ample.

'Cancer and Nutrition: The Positive Scientific Evidence'

Cancer Help Centre nutrition database author Dr Sandra Goodman and I have prepared a booklet with the above title, containing a brief summary of the scientific evidence for giving vitamins and minerals in cancer prevention and treatment. This may be useful to help persuade you of the validity of this approach and to help encourage doctors to prescribe these substances for those with cancer. This booklet is available from the Bristol Cancer Help Centre for £5.00 + £1 post & packing, payable in advance. Access to the nutrition database is also available to all.

CONCLUSION

I hope that now having read this book you will feel sufficiently convinced, informed and inspired to set about changing the way you eat, confident that this can cause a really good creative and exciting change in your life and health. I hope that you feel encouraged to make the change in a gentle, exploratory way without stressing yourself or making yourself unhappy in the process.

I can assure you that, since starting to work at the Cancer Help Centre our catering consultant, Jane Sen has demonstrated beyond a shadow of doubt that vegan cookery can be just as delicious and glamorous as any other form of food. Indeed, she has created a whole new style of cuisine from her work with this approach, called *cuisine vivante*. I now take great pleasure in referring you on to her book, *Healing Foods Cookbook*, which will give you all the inspiration, instruction and ideas you need to make the change.

Play, experiment and become convinced yourself of the real potential for delighting yourself with this way of cooking and eating, and enjoy the satisfaction and deep healing process which comes from properly nurturing yourself as you become fit, healthy, happy and strong.

Glossary

allergen	substance promoting an allergic reaction
angina	heart pain caused by lack of oxygen in the heart muscle, normally caused by narrowing of the heart's arteries
antioxidant	substance which retards deterioration by oxidation, especially of oils, fats and foods
cancer promoter	increases cancer cell activity once already cancerous
caprilic acid	weak acid used to help acidify the body to prevent the growth of yeasts such as candida albicans
co-factors	chemicals required to promote the activity of another chemical (e.g. vitamins)
DNA	deoxyribonucleic acid, the main constituent of the chromosomes of all organisms
electrical polarization	presence of an electrical charge gradient
enzymes	proteins produced by living cells which act as catalysts in biochemical reactions such as digestion and metabolism

essential fatty acids	fatty acids which are essential for and are not synthesized by the body
gamma irradiation	irradiation of food with gamma rays, which are electromagnetic rays of shorter wavelength and higher energy than X-rays
hormone-dependent	cancer whose growth is promoted by the presence of hormones
hydrocarbon	any organic compound containing only hydrogen and carbon
hydrogenated fatty acids	fatty acids with an hydroxyl unit attached (i.e. oxygen/hydrogen unit); they are unstable and potentially disruptive to the body
initiator	starts off cancer cell development
kilojoule	measure of energy equal to 1,000 joules
malabsorption	imperfect or defective absorption of nutrients through the gut wall
metabolize	referring to the chemical process which occurs in living organisms resulting in growth, energy production, waste elimination, etc.
oxidative damage	damage to tissues and biochemical processes via free radicals
phytochemical	plant chemical
salt petre	potassium nitrate, used to preserve meat
transmembrane potential	an electrical charge gradient on two sides of a cell membrane

References

CHAPTER ONE

1. Office of Population Censuses & Surveys
2. Chronic Diseases Control Branch, Bal & Forrester, *Cancer* 72 (3 DSuppl): 1005–10
3. Junshi Chen, T. Colin Campbell, Li Junyao, and Richard Petto, *A diet lifestyle and mortality in China* (Ithaca, NY: Cornell University Press, 1990)
4. Dr Margaret Thorogood, *British Medical Journal* 308 (28th June 1994): 6945
5. London School of Tropical Hygiene, *British Medical Journal* June 1994
6. J. Westin, and E. Richter, 'The Israeli Breast Cancer Anomaly', *Annals New York Academy of Sciences*, 609 (1990): 269–79
7. Professor David Orr, c/o The Schumacher Society, Bideford, Devon, UK
8. Thorogood, *BMJ* 308: 6945
9. Office of Population Censuses & Surveys
10. Office of Population Censuses & Surveys
11. Chronic Diseases Control Branch, Bal & Forrester: 1005–10

CHAPTER 3

1. Office of Population Censuses & Surveys

CHAPTER 4

1. (a) W. J. Blot *et al.*, 'Nutrition intervention trials in Linxian (Supplementation with specific vitamin/mineral combinations, cancer incidence and disease specific mortality in the general population)', *Journal National Cancer Institute* 85.18 (September 15, 1993): 1483–92; (b) J. Y. Li *et al.*, 'Nutrition trials in Linxian (Multiole vitamin/mineral supplementation, cancer incidence, and disease-specific mortality among adults with esophageal dysplasia)', *Journal of the National Cancer Institute* 85.18 (September 15, 1993): 1492–98

2. Dr Sandra Goodman, *Nutrition and Cancer: State of the Art* (London: Green Library Publications, 1995)

3. Ferrari, *Biochem. e. Biophys. Acta* 1007 (1989): 3035

4. (a) Dr Rosy Daniel and Dr Sandra Goodman, 'Cancer and Nutrition: The Positive Scientific Evidence', Bristol Cancer Help Centre, July 1994; (b) Nutrition Database, Bristol Cancer Help Centre, July 1993

5. *Lancet* (review article) 347 (January 1996): 249

6. Dr Sandra Goodman, *Vitamin C: The Master Nutrient* (Keats Publishing Inc., 1991)

7. Nutrition Database, Bristol Cancer Help Centre, July 1993

8. Ibid.

9. W. V. Judy, J. H. Hall, W. Dugan, P. D. Toth and Karl Folkers, 'Coenzyme Q10 reduction of adriamycin cardio-toxicity', in Karl Folkers and Y. Yamamura (eds), *Biochemical and Clinical Aspects of Coenzyme Q10*, vol.4 (Amsterdam: Elsevier, 1984).

10. Nutrition Database, Bristol Cancer Help Centre, July 1993; Michael Lerner, *Choices in Healing* (Cambridge, MA: MIT Press): 234, 235.

11. Lockwood, Moesgaard, Hanioka and Folkers, 'Partial and complete regression of breast cancer in patients in relation to dosage of coenzyme Q10, antioxidant vitamins and fatty acids', *Biochemical & Biophysical Research Communication* March 30th, 1994

Bibliography and Further Reading

SCIENTIFIC

Daniel, Dr Rosy and Goodman, Dr Sandra, 'Cancer and Nutrition: The Positive Scientific Evidence' (Bristol Cancer Help Centre)

Flytlie, Dr Knut and Madsen, Bjorn F, 'Q10 – Body Fuel: The natural way to a healthier body – and a longer life' (Denmark: Nφrhaven rotation A/S)

Goodman, Dr Sandra, *Vitamin C: The Master Nutrient* (Keats Publishing)

Goodman, Dr Sandra, *Nutrition and Cancer: State of the Art* (Green Library Publications)

COOKERY

Elliot, Rose, *The Bean Book* (Thorsons)

Elliot, Rose, *Not Just a Load of Old Lentils* (Thorsons)

Gann, Paola, *Italian Vegetarian Cookery* (Optima)

Hom, Ken, *Ken Hom's Vegetarian Cookery* (BBC Books) (Chinese Cookery)

Jaffrey, Madhur, *Eastern Vegetarian Cooking* (Jonathan Cape)

Jaffrey, Madhur, *Indian Cookery* (BBC Books)
    (not exclusively vegetarian)
Kenton, Lesley, *Raw Energy Recipes* (Vermilion)
Leneman, Leah, *Simply Vegan* (Thorsons)
Ross, Janet, *Leaves from Our Tuscan Kitchen* (Penguin)
Sen, Jane, *Healing Foods Cookbook* (Thorsons)
Wakeman, Alan, *The Vegan Cookbook* (Faber & Faber)

Index